PUBLIC LIBRARY

This book is a perfect prescription for a h[...] biblical health principles and then reveals how evidence-based science has reached the same conclusions. This book will transform your body, mind, and soul. Read it!

—David Stevens, MD, MA (Ethics)
Chief executive officer,
Christian Medical and Dental Associations

Spiritual Secrets to a Healthy Heart is a complete, comprehensive guide for all of us to apply the principles of the Holy Bible to live a healthier life. Heart disease, even though it does not get the fanfare of "the big C" (cancer), is the number one killer of women, and this book explains the relevance of this disease and numerous ways we can stop it from being our fate.

—Bonnie Mechelle
Executive producer of Healthtopia Radio
Creator of the Victory Steps Christian Weight-Loss
Program

Dr. Davis wonderfully addresses the inseparable nature of one's spirit, mind, and body. Her knowledge of both medical facts and spiritual truths recorded in the Bible coupled with her devotion to God and love of people makes this book a must-read for those who desire to care for their physical heart.

—Dale Fletcher, MS
Founder, Faith and Health Connection

God wants us to be healthy. He has given us much wisdom in the Bible and through scientific investigation in how to live a healthy lifestyle. But it is up to us to apply this wisdom to our daily life. In this well-researched and documented book on healthy living Dr. Davis combines physical, emotional, relational, and spiritual components of health and of the causes of many diseases, with special emphasis on coronary artery disease. She provides many practical guidelines on how to live, eat, work, and play well in order to enjoy the healthy life God intends for us. This is biblical and scientific wholism at its best and in a highly readable, sensible, and pragmatic style. Putting into practice this wealth of information will strengthen your heart and add productive and tasty years to your life.

—DANIEL E. FOUNTAIN, MD, MPH
FACULTY MEMBER, CHRISTIAN MEDICAL AND DENTAL
ASSOCIATIONS' CONTINUING MEDICAL EDUCATION PROGRAM

You will never look at the Bible the same way again. It was right there all along—the gospel of health. Everything we need to live a healthy and fit life is captured in the *Spiritual Secrets to a Healthy Heart* by Dr. Kara Davis, with scientific examples supporting the Scriptures. Finally we can no longer ignore the interdependence of body, mind, and spirit in order to live life to its fullest. My heart leaps for joy!

—ETTA DALE HORNSTEINER
AUTHOR OF *THE TEN COMMANDMENTS*
FOR LIVING A HEALTHY AND FIT LIFE

According to Matthew 12:34, "Out of the abundance of the heart, the mouth speaks." What an appropriate observation to describe *Spiritual Secrets to a Healthy Heart* by Dr. Kara Davis. She has challenged the reader with God's Word to support her scientific claims of how we live, how we feel, and how it is! If you desire an appetizing manuscript that will bless you spiritually and motivate you physically, Dr. Davis's work is a must-read. It has the capacity to add years to your life and life to your years!

—GLENDA F. HODGES, PhD, JD, MDiv
DIRECTOR, SPIRITUALITY IN MEDICINE
HOWARD UNIVERSITY HOSPITAL, WASHINGTON DC

As a book linking cardiovascular problems and nutrition, this book is a must-read. Dr. Davis has identified the important aspects of this paradigm and unearthed refreshing information understandable by all who read this book.

—HAROLD B. BETTON, MD, PhD
ASSISTANT PROFESSOR,
DEPARTMENT OF FAMILY AND COMMUNITY MEDICINE
HOWARD UNIVERSITY, WASHINGTON DC

SPIRITUAL SECRETS
to a
Healthy Heart

KARA DAVIS, MD

SILOAM

Most Charisma House Book Group products are available at special quantity discounts for bulk purchase for sales promotions, premiums, fund-raising, and educational needs. For details, write Charisma House Book Group, 600 Rinehart Road, Lake Mary, Florida 32746, or telephone (407) 333-0600.

Spiritual Secrets to a Healthy Heart by Kara Davis, MD
Published by Siloam
Charisma Media/Charisma House Book Group
600 Rinehart Road
Lake Mary, Florida 32746
www.charismahouse.com

This book or parts thereof may not be reproduced in any form, stored in a retrieval system, or transmitted in any form by any means—electronic, mechanical, photocopy, recording, or otherwise—without prior written permission of the publisher, except as provided by United States of America copyright law.

Unless otherwise noted, all Scripture quotations are from the New King James Version of the Bible. Copyright © 1979, 1980, 1982 by Thomas Nelson, Inc., publishers. Used by permission.

Scripture quotations marked amp are from the Amplified Bible. Old Testament copyright © 1965, 1987 by the Zondervan Corporation. The Amplified New Testament copyright © 1954, 1958, 1987 by the Lockman Foundation. Used by permission.

Scripture quotations marked kjv are from the King James Version of the Bible.

Scripture quotations marked nas are from the New American Standard Bible, copyright © 1960, 1962, 1963, 1968, 1971, 1972, 1973, 1975, 1977, 1995 by The Lockman Foundation. Used by permission. (www.Lockman.org)

Scripture quotations marked niv are from the Holy Bible, New International Version. Copyright © 1973, 1978, 1984, International Bible Society. Used by permission.

Cover design by Nathan Morgan
Design Director: Bill Johnson
Author photograph by Karen Forsythe Photography

Copyright © 2013 by Kara Davis, MD
All rights reserved

Visit the author's website at www.drkaradavis.com

Library of Congress Cataloging-in-Publication Data
Davis, Kara.
 Spiritual secrets to a healthy heart / Kara Davis. -- 1st edtion.
    p. cm.
 Includes bibliographical references and index.
 ISBN 978-1-61638-464-7 (trade paper) -- ISBN 978-1-62136-023-0
(ebook)
 1. Health--Religious aspects--Christianity. 2. Spirituality--Health
aspects. I. Title.
 BT732.D38 2013
 248.4--dc23
                                    2012043123

This book contains the opinions and ideas of its author. It is solely for informational and educational purposes and should not be regarded as a substitute for professional medical treatment. The nature of your body's health condition is complex and unique. Therefore, you should consult a health professional before you begin any new exercise, nutrition, or supplementation program or if you have questions about your health. Neither the author nor the publisher shall be liable or responsible for any loss or damage allegedly arising from any information or suggestion in this book.

The statements in this book about consumable products or food have not been evaluated by the Food and Drug Administration. The publisher is not responsible for your specific health or allergy needs that may require medical supervision. The publisher is not responsible for any adverse reactions to the consumption of food or products that have been suggested in this book.

While the author has made every effort to provide accurate telephone numbers and Internet addresses at the time of publication, neither the publisher nor the author assumes any responsibility for errors or for changes that occur after publication.

First edition

13 14 15 16 17 — 9 8 7 6 5 4 3 2 1
Printed in the United States of America

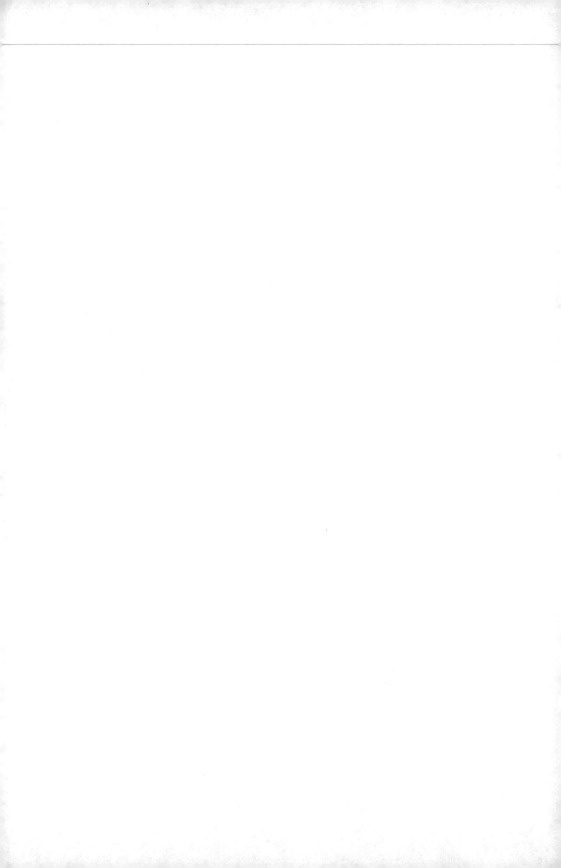

To Lance: My husband, my pastor, my best friend … my heart

Contents

PART II
HOW WE FEEL

PART III
HOW IT IS

Acknowledgments

NUMEROUS PEOPLE CONTRIBUTED TO THIS PROJECT IN ONE way or another—many who were unaware that they were even a source of help. I am grateful for each of them. I am especially indebted to my editor, Jevon Bolden, who was the first to catch the vision and felt confident that I was God's vessel to bring it to pass; thanks for believing in me. A great big "group hug" goes to the Health Team of New Zion Christian Fellowship Covenant Church. These men and women serve the Lord in a fervent way and always place the needs of others above their own. Thank you for your friendship and for being a constant source of encouragement. It goes without saying that my husband, Lance Davis, means more to me than words can possibly express. I am honored to be his wife. In all things (writing included) our four children—Grace, Andrew, Lance, and Natalie—have helped me keep my focus on the "big picture," on things that are truly important rather than minor distractions.

Throughout my life my mother, Eura Foster, has been a source of unconditional support for my sisters and me. For this work especially she has been a source of inspiration by refusing to let a little coronary artery disease slow her down. When I was a little girl, my father, Walter Thomas, planted the seed in my soul to follow in the footsteps of his father and pursue a career in medicine. Thank you, Daddy. My mother-in-law, Phyllis Davis, is indeed my Naomi. I am so grateful that she introduced me to the riches found in God's Word and instilled in me a passion to study it. Andrew Davis III, my late father-in-law, was a man of wisdom, integrity, and kindness whom we all sorely miss. I am thankful for his legacy, which my husband and I have passed on to our children. He would have been so proud of me.

Finally, a special shout-out to all the patients who have touched my life over the years. I have gained so much more from them than they could have possibly gained from me. Thanks a million!

Introduction

My son, pay attention to what I say; listen closely to my words. Do not let them out of your sight, keep them within your heart; for they are life to those who find them and health to a man's whole body. Above all else, guard your heart, for it is the wellspring of life.

Proverbs 4:20–23, NIV

"GUARD YOUR HEART." IF YOU ASKED ME TO LIST THE THEME for this book, or my purpose for writing it, I would quote that phrase from Solomon's writings. In this passage the wise king is speaking to his son. Like any good parent he diverges momentarily to ask, "Are you listening?" From the very first chapter Solomon has presented his son with a wealth of life-preserving information. Now he pauses to confirm that his words have an attentive ear, counseling, "Above all else, guard your heart."

Solomon spoke primarily of the figurative heart—the part of our being some refer to as the "soul" or "spirit." However, here he points out an additional blessing, noting that wisdom will impart "health to a man's *whole* body" (emphasis added). Yes, wisdom blesses our spirit-man, but the benefits encompass our physical, mental, and emotional health. God's Word and godly wisdom will keep us whole in body, soul, and spirit.

In order to appreciate this, we have to make sure we grasp a proper concept of wholeness. We have a tendency to look at ourselves as separate parts that are fit together to make one unit, much like a jigsaw puzzle.

With such a mind-set we approach our health (and life itself) in a fragmented fashion. I see my doctor for my "physical" piece, attend a worship service for the "spiritual" piece, and go to the spa or practice yoga to benefit my "mental and emotional" piece. However, we do not resemble a jigsaw puzzle. We are more like clay, made up of a variety of substances, including minerals, organic material, and water. Yet these separate components mesh together and blend smoothly into one homogeneous substance.

The Bible confirms this when the apostle Paul (from now on I will just use "Paul") describes us as "earthen vessels" (2 Corinthians 4:7). In his distress Job pleaded to God, "Remember, I pray, that You have made me like clay" (Job 10:9). In the eighteenth chapter of Jeremiah God told the prophet to visit a house of pottery to see a tangible example of how we resemble clay in His hands. Like a modern marvel we are separate yet inseparable, created with distinct components. They blend into one entity, housed inside our physical body. So what affects one *part* of our being (whether spiritual, physical, mental, or emotional) affects our *entire* being.

This is a book about the heart—the physical heart and its health. But using the analogy of clay as a backdrop, I will examine the issue of heart disease with the understanding that our physical health is inextricably linked with our spiritual, mental, and emotional health. This is similar to the approach taken with obesity and overweight conditions in my earlier book, *Spiritual Secrets to Weight Loss*.

The Format

Spiritual Secrets to a Healthy Heart is divided into three parts:

In Part 1, "How We Live," I address modifiable risk factors for heart disease. These are things within our power to change, such as diet, weight, activity level, and bad habits like tobacco and excessive alcohol use. This section includes information that has been proven by medical studies. In addition to scientific data, I will provide examples of how science often confirms what the Bible has said all along. Although being obese or overweight poses risk factors for heart disease, I will not cover weight loss in detail. Instead I will focus on the role of weight in heart disease. Though I am biased, I highly recommend *Spiritual Secrets to Weight Loss* for anyone interested in a biblical approach to this topic.

Part 2, "How We Feel," covers the connection between heart disease and mental health. It examines the role of depression and stress from both a medical and a biblical standpoint. I also discuss emotions, including the benefits of positive emotions and the consequences of harboring such toxic feelings as anger, bitterness, and envy. I must note that it is difficult to employ a scientific approach to study the connection between emotions and heart disease; our feelings are not "hard data." Unlike such risk factors as high blood pressure and high cholesterol, emotions are neither tangible nor easy to measure. Therefore there is not nearly as much medical data on the role of emotions. Still, we cannot ignore what the Bible teaches about their impact on our health. This section will examine these biblical precepts.

In Part 3, "How It Is," I review the grim truth we have a tendency to overlook: disease, disability, and death entered the world with the fall of mankind. As long as we are here, we will have to contend with this reality. Our bodies are the temples of the Holy Spirit, so we should feel compelled—even obligated—to do all we can to promote and preserve good health for ourselves and our families. Yet we do this with an awareness that some things that negatively affect health are beyond our ability to control. In the case of heart disease, this includes the process of aging, gender, and a genetic predisposition.

This last section provides an overview of the medications available for treating heart disease, specifically ones used to treat risk factors of high blood pressure (hypertension) and high cholesterol (hyperlipidemia or dyslipidemia). It will also cover the steps that are possible beyond taking pills and look at some of the more invasive approaches used to restore circulation to clogged arteries.

The Problem

"Heart disease" is a generic term that needs clarification. For starters, any number of disorders can afflict the heart, including infections, malignancies, and autoimmune disease. In general, when speaking of heart disease I am not referring to these. Additionally, the heart may not function properly as a result of conditions that originate in other parts of the body—for example, severe anemia and thyroid diseases. I am not referring to this category either. The heart is a structurally complex organ. Some people are born with congenital defects that distort their heart's "architecture." Others have problems with specific areas within the heart, such as the valves or tissue that envelops it—known as the pericardium. Once again I am generally not referring to these as "heart disease."

With that said, what exactly do I mean? Generally, those conditions more precisely termed "coronary heart disease." The source of this problem is atherosclerosis lining the heart's arteries and limiting the circulation (hence the term "clogged arteries"). However, the body contains arteries everywhere, not just in the heart. So coronary heart disease is really a subset of a broader category of diseases known collectively as "cardiovascular disease" (CVD). The umbrella of CVD is made up of four categories that include arteries throughout the body. It is common, affecting the majority of adults over sixty years of age. Coronary heart disease (CHD) is the most common of the four manifestations of cardiovascular disease, making up about one-third to one-half of all cases. There are four manifestations of coronary heart disease:

Myocardial infarction: This is the medical term for a heart attack. The blood supply to a portion of the heart muscle (myocardium) is reduced to the extent that the tissue dies (infarction) because of a lack of oxygen, which is carried by the bloodstream. The blood supply is reduced because of blockage in the arteries in the form of a clot (known as a "thrombus") and, in some cases, from artery spasms. Clots form inside the arteries when areas containing excessive amounts of cholesterol buildup (cholesterol plaques) break or rupture.

Angina: Stable angina (or chronic stable angina) is the sensation of chest discomfort with physical activity or mental or emotional stress. It is predictable and can be relieved by rest or nitroglycerine tablets. Stable angina usually lasts only a few minutes and does not permanently damage the heart muscle. However, unstable angina is unexpected and may occur at rest. It is typically more severe, lasts longer, and poses a medical emergency. Left unchecked, unstable angina can lead to a myocardial infarction or cardiac arrest.

Heart failure: Damaged heart muscle is not able to contract with as much force and strength as a healthy heart. As a result, it does not pump blood efficiently. This results in fatigue, shortness of breath, and difficulty with walking, climbing stairs, and carrying out everyday activities.

Sudden cardiac death: Myocardial infarction is caused by a blockage in the circulation, but sudden cardiac death results when the heart's electrical system malfunctions, leading to cardiac arrest. When the heart develops abnormal rhythm, it beats in a chaotic manner and stops pumping blood. For some people this is the first manifestation of heart disease.

According to the 2010 Heart Disease and Stroke Statistics update of the American Heart Association, 17.6 million people in the United States have coronary heart disease, including 10.2 million with angina pectoris and 8.5 million with myocardial infarction.[1] Cardiovascular disease is the number one cause of death in the United States, claiming more lives annually than all cancers combined. It is also the number one cause of death in women, although only about 55 percent of women are aware of this; many still consider it a "man's disease." In recent years the medical community has initiated efforts to increase women's awareness of heart disease and its risk factors, including the "Go Red for Women" campaign (www.goredforwomen.org) that the American Heart Association launched in 2004.

I believe one of the reasons women are not as cognizant of heart disease as we should be is because—unlike *cancer*—it is not a "passionate" disease. When we hear the word cancer, a myriad of emotions churn inside us, such as fear, anxiety, and depression. If I told you, "Aunt Jane was just diagnosed with breast cancer," your gut response would likely be much different than if I said, "Aunt Jane just had a heart attack." Yes, we would feel pretty bad about Aunt Jane's heart attack, but chances are we wouldn't feel distress deep down in our souls. At least, not as much as if the diagnosis was "The Big C." While I am in no way minimizing the seriousness of cancer, the reality is that heart disease poses a far greater threat to the average woman's health and lifespan. The same holds true for men.

Spiritual Secrets to a Healthy Heart will examine the many risk factors for heart disease. As I mentioned, some risks are beyond our ability to control. I will look at age, gender, and genetics but focus more on the risks we can change (at least to some degree) through lifestyle modification. For example, there are tools available to calculate your ten-year risk for having a heart attack or dying from heart disease. The websites for The American Heart Association (the "Heart Attack Risk Calculator," https://www.heart.org/gglRisk/main_en_US.html) and the National Heart, Lung, and Blood Institute (http://hp2010.nhlbihin.net/atpiii/calculator.asp?usertype=prof) have easy-to-use calculators.

The goal is to heed Solomon's advice and guard our hearts. We can do this by adapting a heart-favorable lifestyle—one conducive to lowering bad cholesterol and elevating good cholesterol, reducing blood pressure, regulating blood glucose through a nutritious diet, maintaining a healthy body weight, and engaging in regular physical activity. Naturally, a heart-favorable lifestyle is tobacco free, supplies adequate rest, and uses alcohol sparingly—the latter with a great measure of wisdom.

Earlier I mentioned the negative emotions of anger, envy, and bitterness. Ridding ourselves of these will treat our hearts favorably. By practicing forgiveness for the sake of God, we can reap the benefits of a heart liberated from the burden to seek revenge and the toxicity of resentment. Finally, guarding our heart requires us to examine our mental health, and without shame. Over the years I have observed that many Christians tend to latch on to the stigma of mental illness, thus resisting addressing mental health—specifically depression. We know from scientific studies that depression has a negative impact on heart disease and diabetes. Ignoring it is harmful. We must overcome denial, let go of erroneous beliefs about mental health, and become proactive in taking necessary steps to guard our hearts.

The Qualifiers

For readers who are health care professionals I feel obliged to issue this caveat: this is not a medical textbook. I have done my best to write in the same manner in which I communicate with my patients—using laymen's terms. I hope my colleagues do not criticize my simplicity but recognize my primary audience is not doctors and nurses but those seeking a clear, basic understanding of good health.

Likewise, my faith is who I am. A few years after earning my medical degree, I accepted Jesus Christ as my Savior. Like Paul, I "am not ashamed of the gospel of Christ, for it is the power of God to salvation for everyone who believes" (Romans 1:16). So while this book contains considerable medical information, I provide it in the context of the Christian faith, which maintains that God "formed my inward parts" (Psalm 139:13), that He is the source of all wisdom (including medical science), and that He is the One who heals. His

Word, the Bible, has insight and answers to all matters, including those pertaining to our health. With that said, let's delve into some spiritual secrets to a healthy heart.

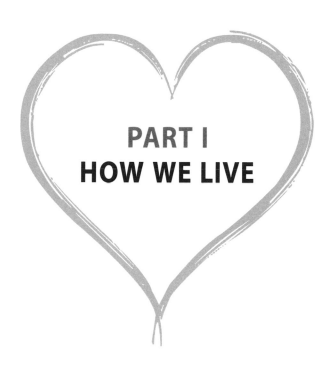

PART I
HOW WE LIVE

Chapter 1

NUTRITION

Oh, taste and see that the LORD is good.

Psalm 34:8

QUICK. NAME YOUR FAVORITE FOOD. CAN YOU FEEL THE smooth texture of chocolate as it melts in your mouth? Savor the burst of sweet juice as you bite into the skin of a fresh peach? Luxuriate in the aroma that wafts from a freshly baked loaf of bread? Food is one of the blessings that sustain our lives. Along with water and air, it represents some of the life-preserving gifts necessary for our existence. Ironically we tend to take these "survival blessings" for granted. How many times have we expressed gratitude for things that rank low on the survival scale? We lift our hands toward heaven to give thanks for a new car, a promotion at work, or a new relationship. Yet at mealtime we only utter a dry prayer—if we even remember to express any appreciation.

In Psalm 34 King David proclaims God's faithfulness and recalls one of many occasions when God spared his life in the midst of dire situations. In the first ten verses he praises God with a heartfelt testimony, using the imagery of food ("taste") to convey His goodness. God's goodness is like a delectable treat—tangible, delightful, and wonderful! Though evident in all aspects of life, His compassion and mercy are clearly manifested through the provision of food. He provides it for survival, enjoyment, and as a vehicle for fellowship.

Mealtimes should compel us, literally and figuratively, to "taste and see that the LORD is good."

In addition to survival, food plays a key role in our strength and well-being. After all, it is not enough merely to exist; we should aim to live life with vim, vigor, and vitality! However, a full life is directly connected to how we eat—namely, the foods and beverages we choose, those we avoid, and the quantities we consume. These three factors have a tremendous impact, especially on heart disease. How we manage them will either optimize or jeopardize our health.

The high prevalence of diet-related diseases in America shows that all too often we make choices that place our health at risk. There are multiple reasons for this:

- ♥ Sometimes we act out of ignorance because we lack understanding of basic nutritional precepts.

- ♥ Other times convenience is the culprit. Given our lengthy "to do" lists, we can rationalize that meal planning and preparation is not a good use of our time.

- ♥ Frankly, sometimes we are driven by our flesh. When governed by our appetites, we will pass up the right foods, go for the wrong foods, and eat way too much of everything.

However, God has given us exactly what we need to conquer these barriers: knowledge to overcome ignorance, discernment to help streamline our schedules, and the fruit of the Spirit of self-control. God has fully equipped us to choose foods that will *edify* our bodies, not *destroy* them. God has done this because He is good.

In Psalm 34 David used the imagery of taste to convey God's goodness. Let's go one step further and consider what tastes might have come to the king's mind as he wrote. In other words, what foods were typical for his culture? What flavors would tempt his taste buds? Since Israel sits on the Mediterranean Sea, the diet of ancient Israelites came from the types of foods now known as the "Mediterranean diet." Over the past few decades much research has been devoted to the relationship between eating and health. While illnesses that come about as a result of vitamin and nutrient deficiencies have long been established, in more recent years knowledge has grown exponentially with respect to how specific food components can prevent disease. This is why the Mediterranean diet is such a hot topic today. There is strong evidence confirming that adapting this eating style can lower the risk for developing many diseases, particularly heart disease.

Of course, Israel is not the only nation bordering the Mediterranean Sea. There are more than a dozen countries along its shores. Each has its own cultural nuances influencing diet. For instance, the cuisines of southern Italy, Greece, and Morocco may incorporate different ingredients and have distinct flavors. Still, there are some key similarities in the manner in which the people from these countries and cultures eat. This manner is quite different from the typical Western diet.

A Mediterranean diet is generally plant-based, consisting primarily of vegetables, fruits, whole grains, beans, nuts, and seeds. Though not necessarily vegan, it features a limited amount of meat, eggs, and dairy products. When these peoples eat meat, it tends to be fish and poultry, with little red meat. It is worth noting that in some Mediterranean cultures the proportion of total fat in the diet is relatively high and may exceed the amount of fat in the Western diet. However, the predominant type of fat is monounsaturated, derived from plants (specifically olive oil) rather than saturated animal fat.[1]

In addition—to use another trendy term—Mediterranean peoples are *locavores*. Recently added to the *Merriam-Webster* dictionary, the word refers to "one who eats foods grown locally whenever possible."[2] Locavores eat primarily whatever foods are in season and therefore are available at local markets. This practice means consuming food soon after it is harvested, with these items containing high concentrations of vitamins and nutrients. While many in the United States think they are riding the crest of a modern wave, in many Mediterranean cultures the locavore lifestyle is a centuries-old cultural norm.

The data connecting this style of eating to better health is overwhelming. For example, the National Institutes of Health's AARP Diet and Health Study included some 214,000 men and just over 166,000 women. Researchers assessed their diets using a nine-point scoring system to measure how closely they resembled the Mediterranean diet. They tracked participants for ten years, with over twelve thousand deaths occurring during the first five years of the study. Researchers found significantly lower mortality rates among those whose diets conformed most closely to the Mediterranean diet, with a 20 percent reduction in death from cardiovascular disease and cancer.[3]

Researchers reported similar findings in a major analysis of twelve separate studies involving more than 1.5 million participants. The composite data from these studies showed that greater adherence to a Mediterranean diet reduced overall mortality by 9 percent, cardiovascular disease mortality by 9 percent, cancer mortality by 6 percent, and the incidence of Parkinson's disease and Alzheimer's by 13 percent.[4]

Many other similar studies across the world show the same results for mortality rates and incidence of cardiovascular disease. What is not entirely clear is the exact mechanism conferring this protection. Is it because the Mediterranean diet causes favorable changes in the lipids, that it reduces inflammation, because of increased levels of antioxidant vitamins and folic acid, or from fiber's beneficial effects on glucose and insulin metabolism? Or a combination of all these factors (and more)? Likewise we cannot overlook the role of other lifestyle variables. People who eat this way are less likely to smoke, more likely to maintain a healthy body weight, and more likely to be physically active—which all play a major role in preventing heart disease.

Finally, it is important not only to acknowledge what the Mediterranean diet *includes* but also to recognize what it *does not* include. Unfortunately the Western diet falls short on two fronts:

- ♥ We are deficient in plant-based foods that are pivotal for good health.

- ♥ We abound with foods that do not have the capacity to protect us against diseases; they may contribute to them.

The first lack is seen by the fact that fewer than 25 percent of Americans eat the recommended five servings of fruits and vegetables each day.[5] Evidence of the latter problem appears via the enormous quantities of foods we consume that are highly processed, made of refined grains, contain unhealthy fats and added sugars, contain too much sodium, and have excessive calories.

When Paul told Timothy that God "richly provides us with everything for our enjoyment" (1 Timothy 6:17, NIV), he spoke in the context of monetary wealth. However, I believe we can extrapolate his words to also refer to food. Truly God gives us food to enjoy. His provisions at mealtime are indeed a source of wealth. They make us rich in sustenance, rich in fellowship, and—if we use wisdom to govern the way we eat—rich in good health. As David said, "Oh taste and see that the LORD is good!"

The Foods We Eat

He causes the grass to grow for the cattle, and vegetation for the service of man, that he may bring forth food from the

> earth, and wine that makes glad the heart of man, oil to make his face shine, and bread which strengthens man's heart.
>
> —PSALM 104:14–15

According to this passage, our hearts (both figuratively and literally) ought to be strengthened and delighted by the foods of the earth. However, this is not always the case. The way we eat is a powerful determinant of whether we will be afflicted by many different diseases, including cardiovascular disease, cancer, type 2 diabetes, and hypertension (high blood pressure). In many respects, what we eat holds the key to our longevity. Ischemic heart disease (cardiovascular disease) is currently the leading cause of mortality in the United States, accounting for roughly 434,000 deaths each year.

Many variables contribute to the onset and progression of heart disease. Still, those related to diet—both the quality and the quantity of the foods we eat—have a tremendous impact. The following table gives the number of deaths from all causes (in thousands) attributed to the risk factors indicated.[6]

Risk factor	Male	Female	Both Sexes
Tobacco smoking	248 (226–269)	219 (196–244)	467 (436–500)
High blood pressure	164 (153–175)	231 (213–249)	395 (372–414)
Overweight–obesity (high BMI)	114 (95–128)	102 (80–119)	216 (188–237)
Physical inactivity	88 (72–105)	103 (80–128)	191 (164–222)
High blood glucose	102 (80–122)	89 (69–108)	190 (163–217)
High LDL cholesterol	60 (42–70)	53 (44–59)	113 (94–124)
High dietary salt (sodium)	49 (46–51)	54 (50–57)	102 (97–107)
Low dietary omega-3 fatty acids (seafood)	45 (37–52)	39 (31–47)	84 (72–96)
High dietary trans fatty acids	46 (33–58)	35 (23–46)	82 (63–97)
Alcohol use[a]	45 (32–49)	20 (17–22)	64 (51–69)
Low intake of fruits and vegetables	33 (23–45)	24 (15–36)	58 (44–74)
Low dietary polyunsaturated fatty acids (PUFA) (in replacement of SFA)	9 (6–12)	6 (3–9)	15 (11–20)

[a]Excludes uncertainty in intentional and unintentional injury outcomes because the attributable deaths used data sources that did not report sampling uncertainty.
doi:10.1371/journal.pmed.1000058.t008

Clearly, Americans have substantial room for improvement for decreasing mortality and preventing disease—especially heart disease. At this writing, debate rages over ways to reduce the burden of preventable disease and thereby curtail health care costs. A discussion on the politics and policies regarding how our country should accomplish this is beyond the scope of this book. What I will address are variables well within each person's scope of influence—the changes we can make as individuals, parents, and families in our refrigerators, on our plates, and inside our cups. When we decide personally to improve our diets, the nation's health will follow suit.

Three Key Categories

Let's turn our attention to three separate nutritional categories and examine how they each affect three of the major risk factors for heart disease: (1) sodium and potassium with hypertension; (2) fat with dyslipidemia; and (3) carbohydrates with type 2 diabetes. I will review these three conditions in greater detail in chapter 8.

Sodium and potassium

Hypertension, or high blood pressure, is the most significant risk factor for cardiovascular disease. It contributes to a majority of deaths worldwide.[7] As the previous chart indicates, it is responsible for the largest number of deaths among US women and ranks second to tobacco use for men. Hypertension appears near the top of lists for diseases impacted by lifestyle. Such behaviors as inadequate physical activity, obesity or overweight conditions, and drinking too much alcohol all elevate blood pressure. However, the greatest influence on blood pressure stems from the presence of sodium and potassium in our diet (both the amount and ratio between the two substances).

Salt has long been known as a major dietary culprit in hypertension. Many research studies confirm the connection between high blood pressure and high sodium consumption. Hypertension appears in about one-third of adults in industrialized countries, where dietary sodium is high. Yet it affects less than 1 percent of people in isolated societies with low dietary sodium, where studies have shown little change in blood pressure problems over the centuries. Yet when individuals from isolated communities move into more urban areas, the prevalence of hypertension increases, along with a steady rise in blood pressure as they age.[8]

Sodium comes in several different forms, which is important to remember when attempting to limit consumption. When I advise patients to reduce sodium intake, the most common response is, "Well, I really don't use the salt shaker" or words to that effect. However, using table salt (sodium chloride) with meals is not the main source of dietary sodium; it only represents about 6 percent of total consumption. While good to keep the salt shaker at bay, the vast majority of dietary sodium comes from processed foods. They contribute an astonishing 80 percent of sodium in the typical industrialized diet.[9] Foods from cans, sealed in packages, inside boxes, or purchased at restaurants contain the bulk of it, even if they don't taste "salty."

While our diets are full of sodium, they are deficient in potassium. This is another consequence of food processing, which adds sodium while reducing potassium and other beneficial nutrients. Our problems also stem from the relatively small proportion of potassium-rich fruits and vegetables in our diets. In the world's isolated communities that follow a natural foods diet, we see the exact opposite: sodium content is low and potassium levels are high. As a result, hypertension is nearly nonexistent.

The difference in the sodium and potassium content in a natural diet compared to a processed food diet is striking. A natural diet provides over 150 millimoles of potassium and about 20 to 40 millimoles of sodium per day. Conversely, an industrialized diet contains 30 to 70 millimoles of potassium and 100 to 400 millimoles of sodium per day. These numbers point to the role excessive sodium and lack of potassium play in hypertension and the relative contribution of these two factors. A natural diet typically has a three- to tenfold higher potassium vs. sodium content. In contrast, the amount of potassium in the highly processed diet typical of the United States and other industrialized countries is generally less than half that of sodium. This is why current research has focused on the *ratio* between the sodium and potassium, not just the *amount*. The evidence is clear that the higher the sodium-potassium ratio, the higher the blood pressure. The lower the ratio, the lower the blood pressure.

Since hypertension is a major risk factor for heart disease, we should not be surprised to find that a high sodium-to-potassium ratio is associated with an increased risk for cardiovascular disease. It is also linked to higher mortality across the board, outside of heart diseases. In a study released in 2011 that analyzed the diets of more than twelve thousand US adults for nearly fifteen years, researchers found that, independent of age, sex, or race, a higher sodium-potassium ratio was associated with a significantly greater risk of death—from all causes, not just cardiovascular disease.[10]

Let's pause to examine the connection between the spiritual and the physical. Consider the verse from Psalm 104 at the beginning of this section, where the psalmist speaks to how God's handiwork meets the needs of His creation. Verse 14 in the Amplified version reads, "He causes vegetation to grow for the cattle, and all that the earth produces for man to cultivate, that he may bring forth food out of the earth." Likewise, in the account of Creation found in Genesis, on the third day, "the earth brought forth grass, the herb that yields seed according to its kind, and the tree that yields fruit, whose seed is in itself according to its kind" (Genesis 1:12). In the seven-day sequence of events, God made sure that the earth produced food prior to days five and six, when He created all living beings that depend on food to survive: "See I have given you every herb that yields seed which is on the face of all the earth, and every tree whose fruit yields seed; to you it shall be for food" (verse 29).

The way God determined we should eat is apparent from these passages, and others. He gave us a predominantly plant-based diet, rich in potassium, with a much smaller amount of sodium. To go a step further, remember how He created our bodies. Psalm 139 gives a poetic account of the way God formed us, with verse 13 addressing the development of our internal organs. He designed them with perfect wisdom, including our kidneys, the organs responsible for maintaining a meticulous concentration of sodium and potassium. From a physiologic standpoint, the kidneys are designed to conserve sodium and excrete potassium. Sodium is maintained in the bloodstream; potassium is secreted into the urine for excretion. This design is absolutely appropriate—perfect, in fact—for a diet containing an abundant amount of potassium and small amounts of sodium.

Our kidneys are "fearfully and wonderfully made" because God created them to precisely match the diet He established for us. However, we decided to switch to foods that are not well suited to the way our kidneys are "knit together." The industrial diet reverses the proportion of these two substances; sodium is abundant and potassium is limited. No wonder we face serious consequences! When we go against God's perfect design, we find that disease, disability, and even death may be the end result.

In order to switch to a diet higher in potassium, we first need to know which foods to choose. At this writing, lawmakers are considering requiring food manufacturers to include potassium content on food labels, just as sodium is already listed. This would allow shoppers to see the amount of each and calculate the ratio in the supermarket. However, the ideal is shifting to foods that don't even need a nutrition label, such as fresh produce and plant-based foods. Whole grains, legumes, nuts, seeds, fruits, and vegetables should occupy a dominant place on our plates. Yogurt and low-fat milk are also good sources of potassium. It goes without saying that eating meals at home and preparing them with fresh ingredients makes a huge difference. With few exceptions, foods served in restaurants and fast-food outlets are high in sodium.

Keep in mind that small changes can make a major impact. Take, for instance, the sandwich you may prepare for lunch at the office or school. While whole-grain bread is a good choice, what do you put inside? For those locked in a "deli rut," the option ends with cold cuts. Those who want to choose better health—and in my opinion, better taste—must broaden their horizons. Using two slices of packaged salami delivers about 560 milligrams (mg) of sodium and negligible amounts of potassium. However, choose 2 tablespoons of peanut butter topped with sliced banana means getting a negligible amount of sodium and about 650 mg of potassium. In addition to the more favorable sodium-to-potassium ratio, the latter is lower in saturated fat. On that note, let's shift gears to discuss dietary fats and the role they play in heart disease.

Fats

Much of what we know about the connection between dietary fat and heart disease comes from the Framingham Heart Study. In 1948 the National Heart Institute (now known as the National Heart, Lung, and Blood Institute) embarked on a major study of cardiovascular disease. Although it had increased to epidemic proportions that long ago, we hadn't learned much about the cause of heart attacks and strokes. So, doctors recruited just over fifty-two hundred men and women between ages thirty and sixty-two from Framingham, Massachusetts. They evaluated participants regularly through physical exams, various tests, and surveys of lifestyle and diet.

Years of careful analysis identified major risk factors for cardiovascular disease, such as hypertension, diabetes, smoking, physical inactivity, and obesity. Even back in 1961 doctors established a connection between heart disease and cholesterol. From the start of the study until today, continuing medical research has expanded our knowledge exponentially. The study is ongoing and now includes some grandchildren from the original group, participants from outside Framingham, and different races and nationalities.

Cholesterol is a fat-soluble substance our body uses in various ways. Incorporated into each cell's outer membrane, it is used to make bile acid (for aiding digestion) and is a necessary component of several different hormones. Cholesterol exists only in animal products—plants don't have any. So quite naturally our bodies would have to be equipped to make cholesterol; otherwise, people would not survive on a strictly vegan diet. Dietary cholesterol contributes only about 25 percent of the cholesterol in our blood; we manufacture the rest internally in the liver.

Cholesterol is a "lipid," a broad category of substances that includes fats and other molecules that are insoluble in water and the bloodstream. Because they don't dissolve, they must link to something that is soluble in blood to be transported to the organs and tissues that will utilize them. Unlike fat, protein is soluble. So our bodies take lipids and bind them to a protein (known as "apoproteins") to form a soluble package that will dissolve in the bloodstream. This apoprotein and lipid combination is called a "lipoprotein." As in all things, the packaging matters; the abnormal metabolism of lipoproteins turns out to be a chief contributing factor to heart disease.

Our current understanding of lipoproteins is complex and growing rapidly. For our purposes, I will focus on two: low-density lipoprotein (LDL) and high-density lipoprotein (HDL). High levels of LDL cholesterol increase the risk for heart disease. HDL, however, has a beneficial effect and actually lowers the risk. This is because HDL transports lipids in the opposite direction of LDL. While LDL deposits lipids in the blood vessels, forming atherosclerotic plaques, HDL removes excess cholesterol from these plaques and delivers it to various tissues (including the liver). There it can be processed into substances like hormones and bile acid. Because of this, a high HDL level is desirable.

So, how does this relate to making a sandwich with peanut butter and banana slices instead of salami? When it comes to improving our cholesterol profile by lowering LDL and increasing HDL, the types of fat we eat matter greatly. Scientific studies have clarified that a high serum cholesterol level plays a major role in heart disease. However, when it comes to which food choices will impact our cholesterol level positively or negatively, we must pay attention to fat—specifically, where that fat comes from and its molecular structure (i.e., saturated, unsaturated, or trans fats). The saturated fats in cold cuts have an adverse effect on cholesterol, while the monounsaturated and polyunsaturated fats in peanut butter have a beneficial effect.

As I mentioned in reviewing the Mediterranean diet, the amount of fat in the diet is not the fundamental problem. The typical diet on the Greek island of Crete derives as much as 35 percent of total calories from fat. Yet cardiovascular disease is less prevalent there than in the United States, where past dietary guidelines recommended fewer than 30 percent of total calories come from fat (more on this later). However, population studies conducted as long ago as the early 1980s confirmed that total fat was not necessarily the culprit with respect to heart disease. Take 1981's Seven Countries Study, which included twelve-thousand-plus participants from various cultures and diets. It found cardiac death rates were not related to *total* fat in the diet but to the percentage of *saturated* fat.[11]

The following table lists the main types of fats, sources, and effects on cholesterol. Keep in mind that fat is categorized based on its major component. For instance, olive oil is categorized as a monounsaturated fat because that is its predominant type, even though about 15 percent of olive oil is saturated fat.

Type of Fat	Sources	Effect on LDL	Effect on HDL
Saturated	Animal products: red meat, whole milk, butter, cheese, ice cream. Plant products: coconuts, coconut oil, palm oil, palm kernel oil	↑	↑ (HDL may decrease when saturated fats are replaced by refined carbohydrates. There may be less HDL reduction when saturated fats are replaced by unsaturated fats)

Type of Fat	Sources	Effect on LDL	Effect on HDL
Trans	Formed by the partial hydrogenation of polyunsaturated fats: commercial baked goods, deep-fried foods, stick margarine, vegetable shortening	↑	↓
Mono-unsaturated	Olives and olive oil, peanuts and peanut oil, avocado, nuts	↓	↑
Poly-unsaturated	Corn, soybean, safflower, and cottonseed oil; fish	↓	↑

If our goal is to optimize health and reduce the risk for heart disease, then we should select foods containing beneficial fats and make every attempt to replace unhealthy fats with healthy—such as peanut butter over cold cuts. Data from the Meat Intake and Mortality Study validate this choice. This study was part of the National Institutes of Health–AARP Diet and Health Study. It included food questionnaires gathered from more than five hundred thousand men and women, ages fifty to seventy-one. Investigators examined the connection between red meat and processed meat consumption with mortality. They found that the risk of death from cardiovascular disease increased as the amount of red meat and processed meat in the diet increased.[12] Red meat and processed meats are high in saturated fat. Unlike the beneficial fat found in peanut butter, saturated fat has an adverse impact on cholesterol.

The Nurses' Health Study produced similar findings. It began in 1976 with nearly 122,000 female nurses. Through the years participants have completed surveys pertaining to lifestyle, medical conditions, and diets. Researchers have gleaned valuable data about women's health in general and heart disease in particular. In one analysis over a fourteen-year span, investigators evaluated the type of fat consumed with the risk for heart disease in some 80,000 nurses. They did not find any significant connection between the amount of *total* dietary fat and heart disease. However, when they looked at specific *types* of fat, they found a striking association. Both saturated fat and trans fat increased the risk for heart disease; polyunsaturated fat and monounsaturated fat lowered the risk. These results showed that *switching* fats lowered the risk of heart disease, rather than *reducing* total fat. In their estimation, replacing 5 percent of calories from saturated fat with unsaturated fat reduced the risk of cardiac disease by 42 percent. Replacing 2 percent of calories from trans fats with unsaturated fats reduced it by 53 percent.[13]

Not only will heart-healthy, unsaturated, plant-derived fats improve the lipid profile, but also their ability to lower the risk for heart disease extends beyond cholesterol. They have other effects that protect the heart. They reduce the tendency toward the formation of blood clots, behave as antioxidants, reduce insulin resistance, optimize the function of the endothelium (thin cells lining the heart), and decrease platelet aggregation.

Notice that in listing some of the ways God blesses mankind, the psalmist said He provides "*oil* to make his face shine" (Psalm 104:15, emphasis added). Isn't it interesting that fats derived from animals (saturated fat) and factories (trans fat, created through partial hydrogenation of polyunsaturated vegetable oil) have an adverse effect on the heart—while fats from plant sources (monounsaturated and polyunsaturated) have a beneficial effect? Saturated animal fat is solid at room temperature; trans fat is a semi-solid. However, unsaturated fats are liquids. So even the Bible reveals the difference between the types of fats. God's heart-healthy liquid fat (oil) makes for a happy face and a happy heart.

Although not all fats are the same, how did the fat-is-bad message become ingrained in Western thinking? Some of the error stems from early versions of Uncle Sam's dietary guidelines, which recommended reducing total fat intake without distinguishing between types of fat. This miscue occurred despite evidence of the differences between fats with respect to cardiovascular disease. Since 1980 the US Department of Health and Human Services and US Department of Agriculture have published the *Dietary*

Guidelines for Americans every five years. In 1980 the "Nutrition and Your Health" brochure offered seven recommendations for good nutrition and optimal health:

1. Eat a variety of foods.

2. Maintain ideal weight.

3. Avoid too much fat, saturated fat, and cholesterol.

4. Eat foods with adequate starch and fiber.

5. Avoid too much sugar.

6. Avoid too much sodium.

7. If you drink alcohol, do so in moderation.

The discussion of recommendation #3 on fat included the following statement: "There is controversy about what recommendations are appropriate for healthy Americans. But for the U.S. population as a whole, reduction in our current intake of total fat, saturated fat, and cholesterol is sensible. This suggestion is especially appropriate for people who have high blood pressure or who smoke." At face value, this implied that total fat and saturated fat were on equal footing and to be avoided. To add insult to injury, recommendation #4 on fiber said, "The major sources of energy in the average U.S. diet are carbohydrates and fats. . . . If you limit your fat intake, you should increase your calories from carbohydrates to supply your body's energy needs."

Even though the government didn't base this "carbs are good and fat is bad" message on solid medical evidence, it remained in the next set of guidelines. In the 1985 brochure, the advice with recommendation #4 said, "Carbohydrates are especially helpful in weight-reduction diets because, ounce for ounce, they contain about half as many calories as fats do." Now we know that this blind replacement of fat with carbohydrates—specifically refined carbohydrates—has contributed to our current obesity epidemic.

Five years later, the 1990 guidelines released with essentially the same seven recommendations. However, this time they used positive terminology, such as "choose" rather than "avoid." It is not clear whether this change in terms helped, especially since so many people have a tendency to "add healthy" rather than "eliminate unhealthy." I see this in my medical practice constantly. Patients are convinced they have made a major lifestyle improvement by adding a piece of fruit to their lunch, even while still consuming a greasy, half-pound hamburger. Choosing right is necessary, but when it comes to improving health, there is a place for avoidance and limits.

In any case, the language changed and the third recommendation about choosing a low-fat, low-cholesterol diet said, "A diet low in fat makes it easier for you to include the variety of foods you need for nutrients without exceeding your calorie needs because fat contains over twice the calories of an equal amount of carbohydrates or protein." Once again, the "carbs are good; fat is bad" message didn't adequately emphasize the differences between types of fats and how they impact our health.

In that same year, recommendation #4 contained the heading, "Choose a Diet With Plenty of Vegetables, Fruits, and Grain Products." While this is great advice, the rationale given for making this choice fell a bit off the mark. It cast fat as an undesirable, even detrimental, category of nutrients: "These foods [carbohydrates] are generally low in fats. By choosing the suggested amounts of them, you are likely to increase carbohydrates and decrease fats in your diet, as health authorities suggest."

The fourth set of guidelines released in 1995 still emphasized reducing total fat, saturated fat, and cholesterol. However, it drew a stronger distinction between the types of fats. It suggested replacing saturated fats with unsaturated and avoiding trans fats. By 2000, with the obesity epidemic in full force, the committee—recognizing its earlier recommendations may have contributed to the problem—included the following statement:

"The committee recommends changing the wording of the guideline to place greater emphasis on reducing intake of saturated fat and cholesterol." From then until now, the guidelines have emphasized reducing only those fats that have been shown to increase risk for disease.

In response to years of misleading fat recommendations, as well as the knowledge that replacing fat calories with refined carbohydrates played a role in the obesity epidemic, an article published in the *American Journal of Preventive Medicine* in 2008 called for a higher standard for future guidelines. The journal said the government should ensure they are based on solid medical evidence rather than opinion or speculation. The authors further advised that when such evidence does not exist, the committee should refrain from making any recommendation.[14]

Certainly the earlier guidelines helped usher in the "low-fat/ no-fat" heyday of the 1980s and '90s, when it seemed producers purged everything of fat to the point of ridiculousness. (Fat-free mayonnaise? Are you kidding?) Unfortunately, while Americans thought we were improving our diets by lowering fat, we did not exchange foods high in saturated and trans fats for those containing beneficial fats. Neither did we switch from saturated and trans fats to foods such as vegetables, fruits, beans, and whole grains. Instead we replaced high-fat foods with "low-" or "no-fat" versions of the same things. Trouble is, refined carbohydrates generally transform "full-fat" foods to "no-fat" versions. So this trend created a surge in our intake of refined carbs. This had a variety of negative consequences: a decrease in HDL cholesterol, an increase in triglycerides, increased body weight, and increased diagnoses of type 2 diabetes, even among children.

Carbohydrates

I don't want to give the impression that carbohydrates are bad; they shouldn't be lumped together any more than fats. Essential to a healthy diet, their significance is confirmed in the Bible passages

I have referenced. However, when the detrimental effects of refined carbohydrates became obvious, popular opinion swung to extremes again. This time it went from "carbs are good; fat is bad" to "carbs are bad; protein is good." Not surprisingly, a deluge of diet plans hit the market that left the impression that carbs were our nemesis and protein our savior. Not true. This category encompasses a wide variety of foods. Some carbs are beneficial; others increase the risk for heart disease, particularly by increasing the risk for type 2 diabetes.

I can understand anyone struggling to understand all the distinctions. It reminds me of when our children were toddlers and one of their favorite television programs featured a segment teaching about similarities and differences. After assembling three or four items, the leader would sing, "One of these things is not like the other, one of these things just doesn't belong, can you tell me which thing is not like the other before I finish my song?" Without difficulty, the three- or four-year-old child playing the game would notice (whether shape, size, or color) and select that item. Imagine playing this game with the leader displaying a loaf of bread, a bunch of spinach, a can of soda, and an egg—three "carbohydrates" and one "protein." Not only would the average toddler be confused, but also so would many adults!

Food categories can get confusing (even to doctors). First, while there are three basic kinds—protein, fat, and carbohydrate—most foods contain more than a single nutrient. Yet they generally get classified based on the predominant one. Even though most people consider eggs a protein, the major component of the yolk is fat. While a loaf of bread contains all three nutrients, it is considered a carbohydrate. There is also confusion arising within a particular category, such as with fats. One type of fat can have a much different effect on the body than another. The same is true with carbohydrates. Barley, kale, and blueberries come under the same "carbohydrate umbrella" as high-fructose corn syrup. Yet the latter has radically different health consequences.

To define *carbohydrate* in simple, chemical terms, it is an organic compound made up of carbon, oxygen, and hydrogen. It is also known as "saccharides" from the Greek work *sacchar*, meaning "sugar." The four types of carbohydrates are monosaccharides, disaccharides, oligosaccharides, and polysaccharides. The monosaccharides and disaccharides are the smaller of the four and are also called simple sugars.

Chemical Name	Common Name	Monosaccharide	Disaccharide
Glucose	Blood sugar	✕	
Fructose	Fruit (plant) sugar	✕	
Sucrose	Table sugar		✕
Lactose	Milk sugar		✕

Oligosaccharides and polysaccharides are made up of more than two monosaccharide units. As such, they are considered complex. Depending on the structure, plant polysaccharides are either easily digestible (e.g., the starch in potatoes and rice) or not easily digestible (e.g., the cellulose that makes up the fibrous and woody parts of plants). Although cows and other ruminant animals can digest the fibrous parts of plants, humans have a limited capacity to do so.

Facts About Fiber

Despite our inability to fully digest dietary fiber, it is a carbohydrate that plays a major role in our health. It impacts our metabolic system (specifically with regard to type 2 diabetes), digestive system (reducing constipation and possibly the risk for colon cancer), body weight, and cardiovascular system. Compared to diets low in fiber, a high fiber intake is associated with a 40 to 50 percent reduction in the risk for heart disease and stroke.[15] For each 10-gram increase in daily fiber, the relative risk for a cardiovascular event is reduced by 14 percent.[16]

There are two types of dietary fiber: soluble and insoluble. Soluble fiber dissolves in water and comes from foods like fruits, vegetables, legumes (peas and beans), and oats. Insoluble fiber does not dissolve in water and comes from numerous sources, including the bran portion of whole grains like wheat, rye, and brown rice. All fiber is derived from plants—hopefully by now you have noticed this chapter's "takeaway" message is to increase plant-derived foods.

While the two types of fiber have different effects, both kinds are beneficial to our health in general and heart health in particular. Fiber has a positive effect on two of the major cardiovascular risk factors: dyslipidemia and type 2 diabetes. Soluble fiber, especially fiber derived from oat products, will reduce the LDL cholesterol (albeit by a modest amount). In one analysis, every 1 gram increase of soluble fiber in the diet reduced LDL by 2.2 mg/dL (milligrams per deciliter).[17] Plus, soluble fiber slows down the rate at which blood sugar rises after a meal, improving glucose control for people with diabetes.

Insoluble fiber also plays a role in reducing type 2 diabetes, with an inverse relationship existing between the two. This is especially true of cereal fiber, which is derived from whole grains. A study involving African American women showed a reduced risk of type 2 diabetes among women who ate a diet high in cereal fiber, whether overweight or not. Researchers concluded that changes as simple as switching from white bread to whole-grain bread, or substituting bran cereal for low-fiber breakfast foods, could reduce type 2 diabetes risk by 10 percent.[18]

The Health Professionals Follow-Up Study and the Nurses' Health Study obtained similar results. They analyzed the diets of nearly two hundred thousand men and women and found that a higher intake of brown rice—a good source of insoluble fiber—was associated with a lower risk for type 2 diabetes. A high consumption of white rice increased the risk.[19] Brown rice and white rice are both rice. However, brown is a whole grain, and white is refined, which brings me to the next point about the wide variety of foods carrying the carbohydrate label.

While both whole grains and refined grains are designated as carbohydrates, there is a big difference between the two. A grain—whether wheat, rice, barley, rye, corn, or any of the many other kinds of grain—consists of three components:

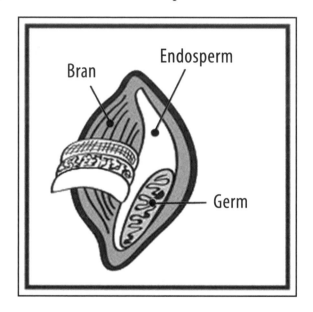

The bran is the outer coating, which contains fiber and vitamins. The germ is the portion containing unsaturated fats and vitamins. The endosperm is the starchy component. The refining process removes the bran and germ, leaving only the white endosperm. This explains why refined-grain products are usually white and why whole-grain products are generally brown, the color of the bran in most types of grain. Since a whole-grain product contains all three components, it is a better source of fiber, vitamins, and beneficial fats than refined. The latter only contains the nutrient-poor, starchy endosperm.

Because of the indigestible fiber content, whole grains contain proportionately fewer calories than refined grains, which may play a role in weight maintenance. Large studies have found that whole grain consumption is inversely associated with body weight. As the amount of whole grain in the diet increases, weight decreases, and vice versa. Beyond body weight, there is an association between the type of grain and body fat distribution. People who eat a higher proportion of refined grains than whole grains are more likely to have central obesity. This means fat deposits in the abdominal area; this "apple" shape (instead of a "pear") represents a fat distribution pattern strongly associated with type 2 diabetes and cardiovascular disease.

In addition, the fiber contained in whole grains has the effect of slowing down the speed of digestion, which reduces the rate of rise in the blood glucose following a meal. The endosperm is starch, and starch is digested easily and rapidly. Think of fiber as a speed bump—you know, those elevations found on some residential streets that force us to slow down for safety's sake. When the starchy endosperm is separated from the fibrous bran through the refining process, the speed bump is effectively removed. So, unhindered by fiber, the starch is quickly broken down inside our intestines into glucose, which enters the bloodstream pretty fast, causing a rapid rise (or spike) in the blood glucose level. When this happens, the pancreas must compensate with matching speed by secreting enough insulin to process that surge of glucose.

In some people this repeated "wear and tear" on the pancreas will lead to the eventual demise of the cells that make insulin, with the end result being type 2 diabetes. In addition to this connection to type 2 diabetes, refined grains also adversely affect the lipids by decreasing the level of beneficial HDL cholesterol and increasing triglycerides. This pattern is associated with insulin resistance, the metabolic syndrome, and cardiovascular disease.

White bread, white rice, white pasta, and the like are all sources of refined grain in our diets. Interestingly enough, another major source of refined grains that we may be less likely to consider comes from high-fructose corn syrup, or HFCS. Derived from the endosperm of corn, a grain, HFCS is now the leading sweetener utilized by the food industry, especially in soft drinks. Introduced in the 1960s, its use spread so widely that it constitutes about 20 percent of total daily carbohydrate intake in the average US diet. Our body weight has climbed alongside this increased consumption. Like other refined grains, HFCS is associated with obesity, insulin resistance, and type 2 diabetes.[20]

The Bread of Life

Without a doubt, the carbohydrate category is the most diverse of the three classes of nutrients in terms of the types of foods and their effects on health. Although the "carbs are bad" concept cannot be applied categorically, this is what happened with bread. Knowledge of some detrimental effects of refined grains fed the notion that bread is a bad food. We embraced this belief so enthusiastically that many fine bakeries, some of which had been around for decades, couldn't weather the storm and went bankrupt.

However, take a moment to consider this from a biblical perspective. Is bread really bad? Is this a food we should shun? If that is the case, how do we reconcile such a belief with these biblical examples:

- ♥ Melchizedek, the king of Salem and priest of God Most High, brought out bread when he blessed Abram (Genesis 14:18–19).

- ♥ Manna, "the bread which the LORD has given you to eat" (Exodus 16:15), sustained the Hebrew nation in the wilderness.

- ♥ Jesus miraculously fed more than five thousand people with five loaves of bread (Matthew 14:13–21).

♥ In describing Himself as the source of salvation, Jesus said, "I am the bread of life" (John 6:48).

♥ Our Lord ate bread with His disciples at the last Passover meal. Then He established the sacrament of Communion with the symbolic breaking of bread: "Take, eat; this is My body which is broken for you; do this in remembrance of Me" (1 Corinthians 11:24).

Clearly bread ought not to have such a bad reputation, especially among Christians! In our quest to reduce the amount of refined carbohydrates we consumed, we threw the baby out with the bathwater. However, it is not bread per se that matters. It is the *type* of bread and the *amount* we eat that affects our health. We need to follow the kind of "eat well; eat less" approach I outlined in *Spiritual Secrets to Weight Loss*. If we govern our appetites by this concept, we will *eat well* by choosing bread made with whole grains rather than refined flour. Then we will go a step further and *eat less* through controlling portions, even with the whole-grain loaf.

This brings us to this chapter's final topic: the connection between body weight and cardiovascular disease.

Obesity and Overweight Conditions

Hear, my son, and be wise; and guide your heart in the way. Do not mix with winebibbers, or with gluttonous eaters of meat; for the drunkard and the glutton will come to poverty, and drowsiness will clothe a man with rags.

—PROVERBS 23:19–21

As I mentioned earlier, during the past several decades our knowledge about risk factors for heart disease has multiplied, along with our ability to treat cardiovascular disease. Between these two advancements we have progressed to the extent that heart disease is no longer the ominous threat that existed at the outset of the Framingham Heart Study in 1948. Yet a steady climb in obesity has undermined these advances by increasing the risk of heart disease.

In adults, obesity and overweight conditions are defined by the body mass index (BMI), a number calculated using a person's height and weight. A person with a BMI between 25 and 29.9 is overweight; over 30 is considered obese. For adults, obesity is further categorized into three levels: obesity I, II, and III. In children, obesity is determined by percentiles. Children at the 85th percentile are overweight; those at the 95th percentile are considered obese. The percentile indicates the number of children in the general population of the same age and gender but who weigh less. While obesity plagues the entire nation, when you look at specific groups, some are heavier than others. People who attend church regularly are at the top of the list.

Researchers have long noticed a connection between obesity and religion. This connection was validated at the 2011 American Heart Association joint conference of the Council on Epidemiology and Prevention and the Council on Nutrition, Physical Activity, and Metabolism, where results from the CARDIA study were presented. This study, which stands for Coronary Artery Risk Development In Young Adults, originated in January 1984 with a group of men and women between the ages of eighteen and thirty. Obviously, they are now middle-aged or beyond.

Information obtained at the start of the study included details on many variables impacting the heart; i.e., diet, exercise, and tobacco use. Researchers gathered other types of information, including religious involvement. They classified religious participation in four categories: high (at least once weekly), medium (fairly regular, but not weekly), low (rare attendance), and never. After eighteen years of follow-up, those individuals with a high level of participation in religious services were 50 percent more likely than those with none to become obese by middle age.[21]

The reasons for this remain speculative:

♥ Is this related to a sedentary lifestyle? Namely, while religious people are sitting in Sunday service, Bible study, and prayer groups, are nonreligious people sweating it out in sports and recreational activities?

♥ Is it related to eating habits? Not only are foods served at a typical fellowship dinner high in calories, but also most people go back for seconds.

♥ Is it because religious people are less likely to smoke? After all, smokers tend to weigh less.

The explanation is not clear, but whatever the case, I hope we can agree that God wants His people to do better. We should show the world how to care for the body, especially since it is God's temple. We should set the standard for a lifestyle exemplified by discipline, moderation, and self-control.

The list of health consequences related to excess weight is exhaustive. Arthritis, sleep apnea, depression, gallstones, asthma, gastroesophageal reflux (GERD), and cancer are all linked to high body weight. It influences the cardiovascular risk factors of dyslipidemia, hypertension, and type 2 diabetes. Aside from the effect of increasing *risk factors* for heart disease, obesity *independently* elevates the risk. This is true even in the absence of hypertension, dyslipidemia, and type 2 diabetes. Multiple studies confirm this, including the Nurses' Health Study involving more than 115,000 women over an eight-year span. In this group, women with a BMI of 32 or above had a risk of death from cardiovascular disease four times higher than for those with a BMI of 19 or less.[22]

As I already discussed, abdominal fat poses a greater risk for heart disease than peripheral fat. And, at least for women, weight gained after age eighteen increases risk, even when BMI is in the "normal" range. Finally, while weight *loss* is beneficial, weight *maintenance* is especially important. The repeated weight loss and weight gain of "yo-yo dieting" can increase risk for heart disease, possibly through reducing the HDL cholesterol concentration with each cycle.

Clearly, obesity and overweight conditions are complex problems and difficult to treat. Without question, the wisest approach is maintaining a healthy weight from birth. This is why measures directed at prevention are at the forefront of health care reform—specifically, preventing childhood obesity. Unless trends change, the next generation will face higher rates of cardiovascular disease and other weight-related illness, more disability, and far more premature death. All of us, Christians in particular, owe our children a better inheritance.

Chapter 2

PHYSICAL ACTIVITY AND EXERCISE

Now behold, two of them were traveling that same
day to a village called Emmaus, which was about
seven miles from Jerusalem. And they talked together
of all these things which had happened. So it was,
while they conversed and reasoned, that Jesus Himself
drew near and went with them. But their eyes were
restrained, so that they did not know Him.

Luke 24:13–16

THE ABOVE PASSAGE RECAPS A KEY EVENT THAT TOOK PLACE
after Christ's death and resurrection. As a detail-driven physician, Luke's Gospel about Jesus's life is lengthier and his depictions generally more descriptive than other Gospel writers. Luke includes incidents in his narrative sometimes not mentioned elsewhere. Or if a story appears in another Gospel, in comparison to Luke's it is condensed. For example, only Mark also refers to the Emmaus experience. His summary covers two verses: "After that, He appeared in another form to two of them as they walked and went into the country. And they went and told it to the rest, but they did not believe them either" (Mark 16:12–13).

I happened to read Luke 24 recently. Although familiar, a truth there captivated me. I had never noticed its significance (which is the beauty of the Bible—it's always fresh!). As I read the passage about Emmaus, I began to wonder: when was the last time I—or any of my friends—set out on foot for a destination seven miles away? Granted, I believe Luke mentions the specific distance because it is his style to include particulars. I am not trying to act "super-spiritual" or read more into this account than Luke intended. Nor do I believe Luke wanted to impress us with the fact these men walked so far. To the contrary, in that era such a distance was unremarkable, just as it wouldn't impress people in many other nations today.

After all, in biblical times walking represented the major mode of transportation. For example, when Jesus encountered the Samaritan woman by Jacob's well, He needed rest because he had just walked about twenty miles. (See John 4.) Nevertheless, I found myself intrigued—so much so that I went online to check the distance for locations I drive to from our home nearly every day. These are places to which I never journey by any means other than a car:

♥ Children's school—4.8 miles

♥ Office—4.3 miles

♥ Church—5.9 miles

What a reality check! These numbers made me painfully aware that as a staunch advocate of physical activity and exercise—and always eager to extol their benefits—I had a short "cut-off" distance when it came to foot travel. Even our church's annual Walk-A-Thon, an event we use to kick off our Fifty-Day Renewal campaign, covers just 3.5 miles. Now, I recognize that the biblical era's culture is vastly different from twenty-first-century lifestyles. If the disciples had access to an automobile, they likely would have driven to Emmaus and picked up Jesus en route.

Still, we cannot ignore the fact that numerous modern diseases directly relate to our lack of physical activity. Researchers estimate that sedentary living is the major cause for approximately two hundred thousand deaths annually in the United States, including deaths from heart disease, type 2 diabetes, and colon cancer.[1] Not only is a sedentary lifestyle an independent risk factor for heart disease, but also inactivity increases the likelihood of developing hypertension and type 2 diabetes. Exercise improves the cholesterol profile, increases the level of HDL cholesterol, and decreases triglycerides, LDL, and VLDL cholesterol levels.[2] In addition, it is nearly impossible to lose weight or maintain significant weight loss without increasing physical activity and exercise.

We don't need to look far to see the burden of diseases related to our sedentary lifestyles. As with obesity and overweight conditions, the evidence is as close as your local congregation. When it comes to moving our bodies, Christians resemble the general population: we are as likely to choose sedentary living as anyone else. Which brings me back to the passage from Luke and another truth worth noting about these men on the road to Emmaus. Not only did they walk with Jesus *physically*, but they also walked with Him *spiritually*. The essence of walking in the Spirit is agreeing with God's teachings and striving to manifest His truths in our daily lives. This is what should distinguish believers from everyone else.

It goes without saying that many lifestyle-related diseases plague the church because we aren't doing enough *physical* walking. However, I would suggest that many of us aren't committed to walking *in the Spirit*. Remember the body-mind-spirit connection means that where we are *spiritually* is evidenced in how we live *physically*. The person who walks in the Spirit leads a highly disciplined and sober life, keeping the flesh under constant subjection. So if we are unwilling to discipline our *physical* bodies, what does that reveal about our *spiritual* lives? Now is the time for each of us to ask ourselves: Am I merely talking the talk, or do I also walk the walk?

With that said, I will review types of physical activity and how physical activity and exercise benefit not only the heart but also the entire body. In general, physical activity can be categorized in three types: (1) aerobic exercise, (2) strength training, and (3) flexibility training, which consists of stretching and warming up. Both aerobic exercise and strength training are beneficial to the heart. While flexibility training is a key element to exercise routines and helps protect against injury, it does not modify the risk for heart disease.

Aerobic Exercise

Do you not know that those who run in a race all run, but one receives the prize? Run in such a way that you may obtain it.
—1 Corinthians 9:24

Whether walking, running, or competitive sports, the Bible contains numerous references to aerobic activity. In the above verse Paul uses the example of a foot race to paint a vivid word picture. He compares the discipline and perseverance of athletic competition to the discipline and perseverance that are a part of true Christian living.

Aerobic means "with oxygen." Aerobic exercise includes activities that use the large muscles of the body in a repetitive, continuous fashion for prolonged periods of time. As our muscles draw oxygen from the bloodstream, we push the heart and lungs toward their maximum capacity—yet without overdoing it. Aerobic exercise includes such activities as walking, swimming, running, and skating. This type of exercise carries the greatest benefits in terms of cardiovascular health and lowers the rate of mortality from any cause.

Strength Training

> She girds herself with strength, and strengthens her arms.
> —PROVERBS 31:17

Proverbs 31 describes the "virtuous woman," who displays noble character and attributes any woman (single or married) should strive to achieve. She is wise, diligent, kind, efficient, and resourceful. An excellent wife and mother, she maintains her home by prioritizing her time and accomplishing meaningful tasks each day. She is also physically fit; according to Proverbs 31:17, her arms were strong. I imagine she had noticeable definition in her muscles, with biceps, triceps, and deltoids that would make any modern-day woman proud. Muscle strength is a benefit of resistance training, but the virtuous woman didn't need to go to a gym or invest in specialized equipment. Her diligence in accomplishing life's routine activities helped her achieve physical fitness. I find it interesting that in a chapter devoted to this woman's admirable qualities, the Holy Spirit includes the fact that she was in tip-top shape. God is interested in our total wellness—not just mind and spirit, but body too.

Strength, or resistance, training is exercises designed to increase muscular strength. It involves working the muscles against a source of resistance. This can be free weights, resistance machines, rubber tubes, the weight of the body (for example, push-ups), or even gravity. Strength training helps to improve metabolism and protect bones against osteoporosis. People who maintain their muscle strength are less likely to fall in old age. Strength training is also beneficial for cardiovascular health, though not as much as aerobic activity.

Active vs. Sedentary

Go to the ant, you sluggard! Consider her ways and be wise, which, having no captain, overseer or ruler, provides her supplies in the summer, and gathers her food in the harvest.
—Proverbs 6:6–8

My objective in this chapter is to convince you that God made us to move. He designed our bodies in such a way that activity is generally more beneficial to our health than sitting around. I say "generally" because there are always exceptions to the rule. There are times when rest and stillness are in order and too much activity is detrimental. Sometimes it can delay the healing process. However, these are exceptions, and we must be mindful to distinguish rules from exceptions. Otherwise, we can make the mistake of validating laziness.

Maybe you have found yourself saying, "I don't want to wear myself out," or "I just need to relax," or "I don't think I should push myself." Is that the truth or a convenient excuse? When it comes to physical activity, the excuses are endless. Many times, if we are honest, we will recognize the root issue stems from a spirit of laziness. Unfortunately, it is quite easy to slip into justifying slothfulness. Proverbs is full of wisdom on this issue, especially in chapter 6, where Solomon advises the lazy person to observe an ant for an important life lesson. I don't know about you, but I would hate to be in a position to need guidance from a bug. That alone should inspire us to shake off our sluggishness and move our bodies a little more!

Activity and Exercise

Before going further, I should clarify these terms. Strictly speaking, "physical activity" and "exercise" are not identical. Physical activity refers to using our skeletal muscles to move our bodies for the purpose of accomplishing things. This can be household chores, transportation (like the men on the road to Emmaus), occupations, or leisure time activities. While exercise falls under the umbrella of physical activity, exercise occurs with the specific objective of becoming physically fit or maintaining fitness. Exercise is planned, structured, and repetitive, but physical activity incorporates random movements as part of daily life. If I devote thirty minutes to walking on my treadmill, this physical activity is classified as exercise. However, when I spend thirty minutes in my yard or garden, I am still engaged in physical activity but am not exercising. On the treadmill, my objective is narrow: physical fitness and better health. In the yard or garden, my objectives are broad: weeding, mowing, planting, and other tasks. While better health is a benefit of gardening, it is not my primary objective. That is why we don't call it exercise.

Physical activity is measured by units called "metabolic equivalents" (METs), which reflect how much oxygen the body uses with a given activity over a certain period of time. When evaluating the intensity of physical activity, the type and time spent are important. Fifteen minutes shoveling snow is roughly equivalent to forty-five minutes of washing and waxing the car. When it comes to overall health, especially our heart health, we have to become "movement minded." Yes, it is important to get the recommended amount of scheduled exercise (which I will discuss shortly), but in this technologically advanced era, it is crucial that we boost our level of total physical activity. We must discipline ourselves to look for more opportunities to move.

There was a time in the not too distant past when we derived physical activity by default. Prior to the Industrial Revolution, people made a living and maintained their homes literally by the sweat of their brow. Life is no longer physically demanding. To the contrary, developed countries feature a pretty sedentary lifestyle. With the invention of modern conveniences (which are upgraded continually), we can accomplish almost everything with ease. Carrying out the duties of our jobs, maintaining our homes, and leisure time activities are far less physically demanding than just a few generations ago.

Even child rearing has changed. Consider how dramatically modernization has reduced the METs of child rearing. In the past a mother had to manually wash every soiled diaper, wring it out, rinse it, and hang it out to dry. If a woman had two or three children in diapers, she could easily burn several hundred calories a day in diaper maintenance. If you compare the METs required to wash and dry cloth diapers by hand with the number required to toss a disposable one into the trash, you can appreciate how physical activity has diminished.

The conveniences of life first ushered in by the Industrial Revolution have dramatically changed our daily energy expenditures. And they are ubiquitous. Though driving a vehicle was never that strenuous, today most cars no longer come with manual transmissions, manual cranks for the windows, or manual steering. TV remote controls are standard equipment (perish the thought of walking across the room to change channels). Plus, remotes used to only change the channel. Now they control the volume, DVD player, Internet, the use of subtitles, and multiple other features. Cell phones and cordless phones have eliminated the need to dash to a mounted wall phone before the caller hangs up. In nearly every aspect of life, we once moved more. Years ago the surgeon general didn't need to recommend the number of minutes per week we should exercise. By and large, people got enough physical activity through daily life. Health and fitness clubs did not gain a foothold until the late 1940s. Ironically, their growth has occurred alongside the development of modern conveniences.

So here's an added problem: we live in an era where a large segment of the population grew up in a sedentary lifestyle. They know no other way to live. Some of us can remember entertaining ourselves with a jump rope instead of television, or playing dodge ball instead of an ever-present video or cell phone game. And though we may have adopted a sedentary lifestyle over the years, active living is not a foreign concept but is something we fondly remember. It is interesting how those of us who are a bit older can reflect on this with a sense of satisfaction—maybe because we intuitively know God created us to move. The challenge, especially for the younger generation, is to first accept that twenty-first-century conveniences mean that routine, daily activities do not meet exercise needs. We must systematically find time and look for ways to move our bodies.

Increasing activity

Unfortunately we can't settle for scheduling exercise during the day. We must also look for ways to increase activity in our daily lives. Believe it or not, this isn't as challenging as it sounds. We simply have to open our eyes for opportunities. They exist in stairways, on sidewalks, in the workplace—even at home.

I remember speaking once to a group of young women who were part of a "Titus 2" ministry. (As an aside, it was indeed a bitter pill to swallow when I realized I was now one of the "older women" Paul mentions in Titus 2:3–5.) Our comprehensive discussion touched on marriage, finances, child rearing, and health. One young woman complained that she hardly had time to maintain her home and definitely didn't have time to exercise. She felt her health club membership was a waste of money because commitments to family, career, and church gobbled up most of her time. Then I put my foot in my mouth. I should have clarified the concept of metabolic equivalents and shown her how daily activities can use the same METs as a health club visit. Instead, I blurted out that she should cancel her health club membership and clean her house. She became visibly offended, and I spent the next ten minutes backpedaling, explaining that I wanted to show her how to kill two birds with one stone. My point: vigorous housework could potentially match any machines at the health club.

Physical activity is beneficial to every part of the body,

particularly the heart. Multiple studies have confirmed that people who are physically fit have a lower mortality rate from all causes of death, not just heart disease.[3] This recognition prompted the release of the *2008 Physical Activity Guidelines for Americans*, which set the following minimum recommendations for children and adults:[4]

Children and adolescents ages six to seventeen

♥ One hour or more of physical activity a day, with the majority of that hour spent in either moderate-intensity or vigorous-intensity aerobic activity.

♥ As part of their daily physical activity, children should engage in vigorous-intensity activity at least three days per week.

♥ Children should do muscle-strengthening and bone-strengthening activities at least three days per week.

Adults ages eighteen to sixty-four

♥ Adults should do one hundred minutes a week of moderate-intensity activity, seventy-five minutes a week of vigorous-intensity aerobic physical activity, or an equivalent combination of the two. This activity should occur in episodes of at least ten minutes, preferably spread throughout the week.

♥ Additional health benefits will come from increasing this to three hundred minutes a week of moderate-intensity aerobic physical activity, one hundred fifty minutes a week of vigorous-intensity physical activity, or an equivalent combination.

♥ Adults should do muscle-strengthening activities that involve all major muscle groups two or more days per week.

Older adults ages sixty-five and older

♥ Follow the adult guidelines. If not possible due to chronic health conditions, be as physically active as abilities allow while avoiding inactivity.

♥ Older adults should do exercises that maintain or improve balance if they are at risk of falling.

Something worth noting is that the guidelines do not mention "low" activity. This is because increased heart and respiratory rates produce health benefits, which only happens with moderate and vigorous activity. Things like cooking, shopping, and simple chores constitute low activity; preparing a meal doesn't typically cause us to gasp for air. Unfortunately many rationalize that low activity is sufficient. When I ask patients how much they exercise, a common response is, "I'm on my feet all day." Well, that's good; it beats sitting down all day. However, if the heart is not pumping any faster or harder, and your breathing rate does not increase, standing a lot does not meet the guidelines' recommendation.

So how do we know if we are engaged in moderate or vigorous activity? One way is to monitor the heart rate to make sure you achieve the recommended target. For moderate-intensity activity, the target heart rate should be 50 to 70 percent of the estimated maximum heart rate. For vigorous-intensity activity, the goal is 70 to 85 percent. So, the first step is to learn how to check your pulse. The next step is to calculate your maximum heart rate based on your age. The third step is to determine what 50 to 70 percent of that value for moderate-intensity activity, or 70 to 85 percent of that value for vigorous-intensity. Finally, you need to monitor the rate to make sure you stay on target. Whew—a bit of a challenge!

Before you throw up your hands in despair, here is the upside to technological developments: some high-tech exercise equipment can perform these calculations. However, while that is fine if you happen to be in a gym, what about swimming in a pool, walking in a mall, or jogging outdoors? Might there be an easier way to determine whether your exercise is vigorous enough without counting and calculating? Thankfully, there is—the "talk test." Generally if you are able to sing during an activity, it constitutes low intensity. If you are able to talk, even in short sentences, but unable to sing, you are engaged in a moderate intensity activity. In a vigorous workout you cannot speak more than a few words without pausing to take a breath.

The guidelines also call for strength training, at least twice a week for adults and three days a week for children. In strength training, exercises work the muscles against resistance while repeating the activity in what are called "sets." The source of resistance can vary and includes free weights, resistance machines, and the weight of the body. All of the major muscle groups should be included—legs, arms, back, hips, chest, shoulders, and abdomen.

Unlike aerobic exercise, which can be done every day, strength training requires a couple of days rest between sessions for muscles to recover.

A Sedentary People

These well-established guidelines are based on exhaustive research and observational studies. The health benefits are far-reaching and undeniable; a considerable amount of data attests to the benefits of exercise. Yet the vast majority of Americans are not even reaching the minimum recommendations. This ought not to be the case—especially when considering the tremendous burden of preventable disease on quality of life, productivity, and skyrocketing health care costs.

Exercise profits our health even when we don't meet recommended daily minimums. In a large study conducted in Taiwan, researchers placed four hundred thousand men and women in one of five categories based on weekly exercise. They included inactive, low, medium, high, or very high. The "low" group exercised an average of fifteen minutes per day (roughly ninety minutes per week), or significantly less than the recommended one hundred fifty minutes per week for moderate-intensity activity. Still, after approximately eight years of follow-up, when compared to the "inactive" group, the "low" group had a 14 percent reduction in mortality and a three-year-longer life expectancy. For those who exercised regularly, every additional fifteen minutes of activity reduced the risk of death by an additional 4 percent. However, the "inactive" group saw a 17 percent *increase* in the risk of mortality.[5]

I recognize that the environments of modern neighborhoods and cities are better suited to vehicular transportation than physical activity. However, I am encouraged by recent efforts in many municipalities to change this through better zoning and development policies. Such regulations require that new developments be more pedestrian-friendly by including sidewalks, crosswalks, more bicycle paths, better signs and pavement markings of existing paths, and including bike racks in public areas and school yards. Even older neighborhoods that are not pedestrian- or biker-friendly are upgrading their infrastructures.

However, what about those who live in environments that inhibit physical activity? While this certainly presents a barrier, a motorized environment is not an across-the-board excuse for inactivity. We can't blame the scarcity of bicycle paths for taking an elevator or escalator when climbing stairs will help us stay fit. The Harvard Alumni Study found that men who averaged at least eight flights of stairs a day had a 33 percent lower mortality rate than sedentary males.[6] Nor does a motorized environment explain circling the lot several times to find a parking space close to the entrance. Or, worse yet, borrowing Grandma's handicapped placard to park right next to the door. Yes, we should become more proactive in removing barriers, but they aren't the only reason for inactivity. The primary one is personal choice.

Researchers have confirmed that we make such choices. In a

study published in 2008, investigators gave more than sixty-three hundred people six years old and older an activity monitor to wear for a week. Participants spent more than 55 percent of their waking hours in sedentary inactivity. The most inactive groups were older adolescents and adults over age sixty; both groups spent more than 60 percent of their waking hours doing little physically.[7]

What persuades us to reject an active lifestyle with all its benefits and choose a sedentary lifestyle that is detrimental to good health? I have pondered this question at length and concluded that it boils down to attitude and knowledge. While some people don't know the benefits, others don't care. Some rationalize that the data gleaned from research doesn't apply to them. Then there are those who just don't want to change. Since I cannot transform a person's attitude, my focus in my medical practice and my writing is to provide information. I hope that by imparting knowledge, I can persuade or inspire people to take the necessary steps—including regular exercise—to optimize their health.

Made to Move

I will praise You, for I am fearfully and wonderfully made; marvelous are Your works, and that my soul knows very well.
—Psalm 139:14

In Psalm 139 David praises God for the miracle that takes place in the secrecy of the womb. God created us—"knit [us] together" is the terminology used in verse 13 of the New International Version—in a marvelous way. You don't need to take a course in anatomy or physiology to appreciate the wonder of the human body. Yet, despite the amazing nature of our bodies, they are not invincible. They require proper, consistent care, including physical activity and exercise. We know that working out and moving more will not make us indestructible "superheroes." However, physical activity will preserve and optimize the "temple of the Holy Spirit" (as 1 Corinthians 6:19 puts it) that God has established.

Exercise's Mighty Impact

Practically every organ of the body functions better with movement. Physical exercise impacts the entire body, especially the heart. With exercise you will see improvements in numerous physical factors, including:

Muscles and bones

Exercise and physical activity increase the strength of our muscles. Strong muscles use energy more efficiently, which is one reason why people who are physically fit experience less fatigue with daily activities. As we grow older, weak muscles increase the likelihood of falling and other accidents; they are associated with a general decline in body functions. Exercise reduces the risk for osteoporosis (brittle bones) and will often reduce the pain associated with osteoarthritis.

Metabolism

Exercise is an essential component to diabetes management. For those suffering from type 2 diabetes, exercise improves glucose control through several mechanisms. One is making our cells more responsive to insulin. The benefits are significant—as good as adding another medication. One of the blood tests used to monitor diabetes is known as hemoglobin A1c. In type 2 diabetics, studies show that at least one hundred fifty minutes per week of structured exercise will improve hemoglobin A1c to the same extent as adding a non-insulin medication. While exercising less than one hundred fifty minutes per week does have benefits, it is not as pronounced.[8]

Exercise also reduces the risk of cardiovascular disease among people with type 2 diabetes. In one study of nearly three thousand diabetic adults, those who walked at least two hours each week had a lower risk for cardiovascular death compared to inactive individuals. The risk was even lower for those who walked three to four hours each week.[9] There is also strong data showing that regular exercise can delay the onset or even prevent the development of type 2 diabetes.

Dyslipidemia

This refers to disordered lipids in the blood—in layman's terms, high cholesterol. Exercise will improve the lipid profile by lowering the triglyceride and LDL cholesterol levels and elevating good HDL cholesterol. The benefits to HDL alone can reduce the risk for heart attack by 15 percent.

Cancer

Regular exercise may provide modest protection against the development of cancers, specifically breast, pancreatic, and colon. Exercise is also beneficial to people who have been treated for cancer. It improves their quality of life and overall rate of survival.[10]

Cognitive function and independent living

Maintaining even a moderate amount of physical activity while we are young will increase the probability of better health and independent living as we age. Studies show that regular exercise delays the onset of Alzheimer's disease and other forms of dementia in older people.[11] These benefits apply both to seniors who are active and able to live independently within the community, as well as those who reside in nursing homes.

Psychological health

Compared to those who are active, depression is more common in sedentary adults. Physical activity, whether low intensity or vigorous intensity, reduces the likelihood of developing depression. Of course, vigorous exercise is more effective.[12] Exercise also eases the symptoms of anxiety and is an ideal stress reliever.

Heart

One of the reasons exercise is so beneficial to the cardiovascular system is that it improves or eliminates many risk factors for heart disease, along with independent positive impact on the heart. I have already discussed the positive effects of exercise on the major risk factors of dyslipidemia and diabetes. Because of its ability to reduce stress and curtail depression, exercise also lessens the detrimental effects our emotions can have on the cardiovascular system. And exercise increases the likelihood for success in smoking cessation, reduces obesity, and improves blood pressure control.

Since breaking a cigarette addiction is a tough challenge, any tool that can assist a smoker in quitting is extremely valuable. Exercise is such a tool. In one study designed to examine the role of exercise in smoking cessation, women who engaged in a vigorous exercise program—coupled with therapy—had better rates of quitting than females who relied solely on behavioral therapy. In addition, women who exercised gained less weight after quitting, a common hazard for ex-smokers.[13]

Weight loss and weight maintenance are nearly impossible to achieve without regular exercise. Aside from weight, another benefit of exercise is its positive effect on body fat distribution. Sedentary people are more likely to have central, abdominal obesity than the physically active. Central obesity features a greater risk for cardiovascular disease, diabetes, and hypertension.

Finally, regular exercise helps lower blood pressure as effectively as some blood pressure medications. It can even help prevent or delay the development of hypertension. Exercise does this by improving the ability of the arteries to relax (meaning they generate less pressure). It lowers the levels of hormones that can increase blood pressure and modifies hormones that control how our kidneys process sodium. Exercise sustains these blood-pressure-lowering effects for many hours afterward. People who maintain an active lifestyle will reap the benefits for years.

The evidence is overwhelming—God designed us for physical activity. Whether the data comes from scientific studies, intuition, or precepts and examples from the Bible, we have abundant proof regarding activity's health benefits. Let's be good to our bodies (especially our hearts) and do our best to move more.

Chapter 3

HABITS AND PREFERENCES

But the fruit of the Spirit is . . .
self-control. Against such there is no law.
Galatians 5:22–23

I N THE FIFTH CHAPTER OF GALATIANS PAUL DESCRIBES MANY attributes of the flesh nature before listing nine characteristics of the Holy Spirit. These fruit of the Spirit include love, joy, peace, patience, kindness, goodness, faithfulness, gentleness, and self-control. I think of the last one as the "neglected ninth." Many of us like to overlook it or at least play down its significance; some wish Paul had never mentioned it. Now, the other eight don't bother us a bit. We can acknowledge imperfections and know there is plenty of room to grow in such qualities as love, joy, and peace. And who can deny that patience is a virtue? Even an atheist sees value in kindness and gentleness.

However, when it comes to self-control, many of us can imitate the prophet Isaiah and cry, "Alas! Woe is me!" We can easily think of careless words better left unspoken, money spent that we should have saved, taking that extra spoonful of sugar, or those secret indulgences. After all, we like "having it our way" in the drive-through lane. All fall under the convicting shadow of self-control (that is, a lack of it). In a culture that glorifies excess and exalts permissiveness, it becomes easy to sell short the importance of this beloved, sacred attribute of the Holy Spirit.

In this chapter I will examine two areas where self-control helps preserve health. The first is tobacco, where self-control will either equip us to never pick up this nasty habit or empower us to quit. The second is alcohol, which requires moderation (the *evidence* of self-control). In both instances forsaking self-control is detrimental to the heart; maintaining self-control will prove beneficial.

Both tobacco and alcohol carry the potential for addiction. However, instead of discussing addiction, I will review the effects of tobacco and alcohol on our bodies, focusing on our hearts. Addiction is real, both physiologically and psychologically, and plays a major role in tobacco and alcohol abuse. My omission does not minimize them. Anyone who has conquered an addiction will attest to the difficulty of overcoming this hurdle. For some it is seemingly impossible. If this is a problem, I encourage you to seek assistance from your health care provider to learn what resources—including prescription medications—can help.

Tobacco

> Or do you not know that your body is the temple of the Holy Spirit who is in you, whom you have from God, and you are not your own? For you were bought at a price; therefore glorify God in your body and in your spirit, which are God's.
>
> —1 Corinthians 6:19–20

In His Sermon on the Mount, Jesus said, "Do not think that I came to destroy the Law or the Prophets. I did not come to destroy but to fulfill" (Matthew 5:17). Under the Law the Israelites built the temple with an inner sanctuary called the "most holy place," located just beyond an area called the "holy place." After completing the building, the priests placed the ark of the covenant inside the most holy place, and "when the priests withdrew from the Holy Place, the cloud filled the temple of the LORD. And the priests could not perform their service because of the cloud, for the glory of the LORD filled his temple" (1 Kings 8:10–11, NIV). The Lord abided in this most holy place.

Jesus fulfilled the Law through His sacrificial death. After His crucifixion and death, "the veil of the temple was torn in two from top to bottom" (Matthew 27:51). The significance: previously this curtain blocked the entrance into the most holy place. When God ripped it apart, He signified that He had opened the way into His presence to all humans. Fifty days later, on the Day of Pentecost, the Holy Spirit manifested Himself to the disciples present (more than one hundred). He filled them with the Holy Spirit and fulfilled the words spoken by the prophet Joel: "And it shall come to pass afterward that I will pour out My Spirit on all flesh" (Joel 2:28). So with the fulfillment of the Law and the prophets, the presence of God moved from a building into our bodies. However, this transfer did not reduce the importance of God's dwelling place. God's followers treated the most holy place within the temple with reverence and respect. We must treat our physical bodies with the same measure of care.

This is the point Paul made in 1 Corinthians. The understanding that our physical bodies are temples of the Holy Spirit ought to be at the forefront of our decisions regarding their use.

This means the Spirit must guide our behavior, including not only our eating habits but also the use of such substances as tobacco. There is no way to sugarcoat or minimize this truth: smoking poisons the dwelling place of the Holy Spirit. I know many smokers. Since I love them, I warn them that smoking is a toxic habit, helps destroy God's temple, and leads to premature death. Self-control is vitally important to resist the temptation to smoke, especially since cigarettes are so heavily promoted. In 2006 cigarette companies spent approximately $34 million dollars *per day* to market cigarettes—in the United States alone![1]

Smoking is our nation's leading cause of preventable death and disability. Every year around 443,000 people die from smoking or exposure to secondhand smoke, while 8.6 million suffer from a serious smoking-related illness. Women appear more susceptible than men to the detrimental effects of tobacco, at least with respect to heart disease.[2] According to the World Health Organization, tobacco causes about 8.8 percent of deaths worldwide. Globally, approximately 4 million people die each year from smoking-related causes. If current trends continue, by 2025 this number is expected to increase to as many as 10 million.[3]

Despite widespread knowledge about the hazards of smoking, it remains a fairly common habit. Currently an estimated 22 percent of men and 17.5 percent of women in the United States smoke, or about 46.6 million people. In addition, they regularly expose 88 million nonsmokers to secondhand smoke. Even though increasing taxes make cigarettes ever more expensive, smoking is more common among those at lower income and lower educational levels. About half of people with a GED smoke, compared to only 6 percent of those with a graduate degree.[4]

Most smokers start before age eighteen, most commonly between ages fourteen and fifteen. There is a reason for the significance of age—typically teens are most strongly influenced by peers, don't have a solid appreciation of their own mortality, and have not fully developed the ability to factor long-term consequences into their decisions. Adolescents begin smoking at a stage in life when they want to "fit in" or win friends' admiration. Yet they do not have the capacity to consider things like their health or finances. (It's a very expensive habit!) So they start smoking with little consideration of its consequences. However, as they mature and come to appreciate mortality and understand consequences, they discover how difficult it is to break the nicotine habit. To make matters worse, adolescents are more prone to addiction because their bodies are highly sensitive to nicotine. That is why marketing cigarettes to teens is so unconscionable.

Since 1964 the US surgeon general's office has issued periodic reports on smoking. In December 2010 it released its thirtieth report, *How Tobacco Smoke Causes Disease: The Biology and Behavioral Basis for Smoking-Attributable Disease*. This comprehensive, seven-hundred-page report includes a wealth of information and highlights the following facts:[5]

- ♥ Any exposure to tobacco smoke is harmful, including secondhand smoke or an occasional cigarette. There is no risk-free level for smoking.

- ♥ Tobacco smoke causes immediate damage, delivering toxic chemicals that rapidly travel from the lungs into the bloodstream and to every organ in the body. These chemicals damage DNA, which can lead to cancer, and damage blood vessels, which can cause heart attack and stroke.

- ♥ The damage to the body increases with the number of cigarettes smoked per day and longevity of this habit.

- ♥ Today cigarettes deliver nicotine more quickly from the lung to the brain. They are far more addictive than in times past.

- ♥ There is no safe cigarette. Low-tar and light brands do not reduce the rate of disease and may hinder a smoker's ability to quit.

- ♥ Quitting at any time and at any age is beneficial. Of course, the sooner the better, but there is never a time where the health benefits of quitting cease.

Smoking accounts for almost $200 billion annually in health care costs and lost productivity. While the average cost of a package of cigarettes (including sales tax) in 2010 was $5.29, the estimated health care costs and losses in productivity *per package* totaled $10.47—and this is a low estimate.[6] Cigarettes cause disease throughout the body, including cancer, lung disease, and, of course, heart disease. Although you may claim this is purely a private matter in a free country, what about those relying on Medicaid or Medicare who need treatment for diseases associated with past smoking? And those medical costs are partially paid by our tax dollars.

The effects on the heart are particularly alarming. Smoking increases the risk of all forms of cardiovascular disease. Not only is coronary artery disease more common in smokers, but also they experience a higher incidence of stroke, peripheral vascular disease, and aortic aneurysms. This stems from the damaging effects on blood vessels throughout the body. Smoking is one of the modifiable risk factors for heart disease. Unlike the nonmodifiable risks we incur because of age, gender, or family history, we have the power to eliminate the risks from smoking. It is an especially hazardous habit for people who have other risks for heart disease, such as diabetes, hypertension, or dyslipidemia. In addition, type 2 diabetes is highly prevalent among people who smoke, with strong evidence pointing to the possibility that smoking may cause type 2 diabetes.[7]

Cigarette smoke accelerates the rate of atherosclerosis, both in smokers and those exposed to secondhand smoke. It damages the blood vessels through many mechanisms:

♥ Smoking changes the lipid profile to "heart unfriendly." It decreases the level of beneficial HDL cholesterol while increasing the LDL and triglyceride levels.

♥ Smoking reduces the elasticity of blood vessel walls, which predisposes them to damage.

♥ Cigarette smoke increases a person's propensity to form blood clots, a process known as thrombosis. Blood clots play a major role in triggering heart attack and stroke.

♥ Smoking impairs the ability of the blood vessels to relax and dilate. This can reduce blood flow and limit circulation.

♥ Smoking produces a state of chronic inflammation, as evidenced by an increase in the level of C-reactive protein and other substances in the bloodstream that are reliable indicators of chronic inflammation.

In addition, smoking activates the sympathetic nervous system, which increases the heart rate and blood pressure. When coronary arteries are diseased, this added stimulation to the heart can be sufficient to precipitate angina. If that weren't bad enough, cigarettes deliver carbon monoxide into our bodies. Carbon monoxide is a toxic gas, exerting its harmful effects by reducing the amount of oxygen that hemoglobin can deliver to our tissues. Illinois, the state where I reside, passed a law in 2007 requiring nearly every house and apartment building to have a carbon monoxide detector installed within fifteen feet of the bedroom. The state encourages residents to regularly check batteries to make sure we are safe from accidental exposure. Yet each puff on a cigarette introduces carbon monoxide directly into the bloodstream—willfully, not unintentionally. Does that strike anyone else as illogical?

As I mentioned earlier, there are always advantages to quitting. This is particularly true of cardiac disease. Heart disease risk diminishes relatively quickly after a person quits. The greatest reduction occurs within the first three years. Especially encouraging is that by the third to fifth year of abstinence, excess cardiovascular risk vanishes. However, quitting is not easy. As addictive as heroin and cocaine, nicotine is the most common form of chemical dependence in the United States.

Still, success is within reach, as evidenced by the fact that 47 million people are now ex-smokers. Some are able to quit "cold turkey"; that approach is fine if it works. However, the majority of people need additional help, which should not provoke embarrassment or shame (even if "cold turkey" folks make you feel that way). Counseling is effective, whether in the form of advice given by your health care provider during a routine office visit or more formal approaches. You may try individual or group therapy, telephone counseling (1-800-QUIT-NOW), or behavior modification therapy.

There are also medications to facilitate quitting. Nicotine replacement therapy comes in the form of gum, skin patches, inhalers, nasal sprays, and lozenges. You can purchase some over-the-counter, while others require a prescription. There are also effective non-nicotine prescription medications, such as Zyban (bupropion SR) and Chantix (varenicline tartrate). A combination of medications and counseling is more effective than either approach used alone. It goes without saying that prayer—personal prayer and others' intercession—and dependence on the Holy Spirit (who equips us with self-control) should form the foundation for whatever method you choose.

Alcohol

> All things are lawful for me, but not all things are helpful; all things are lawful for me, but not all things edify. Let no one seek his own, but each one the other's well-being.
> —1 Corinthians 10:23–24

The matter of drinking alcohol is a complex topic from any perspective—medical, social, or spiritual. While the answer for whether or not a person should smoke cigarettes is a categorical no, things are not as clear-cut when it comes to if, when, and how much one should drink. In this section I will examine the potential benefits as well as the risks to the heart with alcohol consumption.

Before delving into the topic from a physical standpoint, consider our responsibilities from a spiritual view. In the above passage from 1 Corinthians, Paul speaks to the issue of Christian liberty.

This topic arises in other epistles, including Romans 6:15, Galatians 5:13–15, and other passages in 1 Corinthians, such as 1 Corinthians 6:12. It was an area of confusion for new Christians nearly two thousand years ago and remains so for many today.

While Jesus makes our liberty possible, Paul clarifies that liberty does not permit us to pursue a no-holds-barred lifestyle. To the contrary, Christ released us from the bondage of sin (as evidenced by our inability to keep the law) and placed us under the full authority and governance (i.e., "the law") of the Lord: "For *the law* of the Spirit of life in Christ Jesus has made me free from *the law* of sin and death" (Romans 8:2, emphasis added). Although Christ set us free, we have a new obligation—serving the Lord. While liberated, we aren't to use our liberty "as a cloak for vice, but as bondservants of God" (1 Peter 2:16).

So, how do we reconcile this truth with the issue of drinking alcohol? As 1 Corinthians 10:23–24 says, we may have *liberty* to drink ("all things are lawful for me"), but drinking may not be a wise choice ("not all things are helpful"). There are circumstances where restricting our liberty is the right thing to do. One is when drinking will potentially cause another believer to stumble. Such a case means alcohol becomes a means of tearing someone down when we ought to build them up ("not all things edify"). This is the crux of the matter. We must avoid drinking if it might hinder another believer or mar our testimony to an unbeliever ("let no one seek his own, but each one the other's well-being").

However, this obligation doesn't end with our concern for other people. Circumstances can prescribe avoiding alcohol, even if drinking alone, including:

♥ If you intend to get drunk, which Ephesians 5:18
  warns against: "Do not get drunk on wine, which
  leads to debauchery" (NIV).

♥ If there is a risk for losing control, whether in terms of the quantity of alcohol consumed or a loss of inhibition in other areas. I refer back to the verse on the fruit of the Spirit that opened this chapter.

♥ If you have a past history of alcohol dependency or substance abuse. As Proverbs 26:11 says, "Like a dog that returns to its vomit is a fool who repeats his folly" (NAS).

♥ In instances where drinking is not wise. For example, if alcoholism is part of your family's history, you are pregnant, or you will need to drive or operate machinery. As Solomon said, "I wisdom, dwell with prudence, and I find knowledge and discretion" (Proverbs 8:12, NAS).

Sadly, although God gave mankind some alcoholic beverages as a blessing, through misuse and abuse we can turn them into a curse. And the capacity for alcohol to bless or curse rests in all areas—mentally, emotionally, and physically.

Potential benefits

> You may spend the money for whatever your heart desires: for oxen, or sheep, or wine, or strong drink, or whatever your heart desires; and there you shall eat in the presence of the LORD your God and rejoice, you and your household.
> —DEUTERONOMY 14:26, NAS

Our natural tendency in numerous situations is to maximize the negative and minimize the positive. Any network or cable news summary leads with bad reports, reserving the "nice" story for the end of the broadcast. However, don't do like the grumblers who love to throw stones at the news media for reflecting human nature. Many of these critics do the same thing—like parents who tend to treat the poor grades on a child's report card as if they were written in neon ink, making the good grades fade by comparison. Or the employers who often need reminders to give credit to their staff for a job well done since they freely issue reprimands and criticisms.

So it is with alcohol. We are keenly aware of such hazards as broken relationships, lost opportunities, sickness, and, in some instances, loss of life. We all know of something or someone destroyed by alcohol. Yet if we look at the matter objectively and without the bias of past negative experiences, we must acknowledge that while alcohol carries potential harm, it includes potential benefits. The Bible confirms this:

- ♥ Deuteronomy 14:26 (which opened this section) comes from a passage of scripture where God instructs the Israelites on how to spend their second tithe. He encourages them to buy whatever they want, including "wine or strong drink."

- ♥ Psalm 104 is a song of praise to the Lord for His provisions. The psalmist acknowledges God as the source of food, oil, "and wine which makes man's heart glad" (Psalm 104:15, NAS).

- ♥ As recorded by John, Christ's first miracle was changing water into wine at a wedding feast (John 2:1–10).

Since God (at least in these three examples) uses alcohol as a blessing, we should not be surprised to learn that light to moderate drinking contains some health benefits, particularly with regard to coronary artery disease and the risk of heart attack. For the sake of clarity, I need to define what this means. A standard drink generally refers to one containing 14 to 15 grams of alcohol, which is equivalent to 12 ounces of beer, 5 ounces of wine, or 1.5 ounces of 80 proof liquor. The following guidelines apply to consumption:

Moderate drinking

- ♥ Women: less than two standard drinks per day

- ♥ Men: less than three drinks per day

- ♥ Elderly (over sixty-five): less than two drinks per day

Heavy drinking

- ♥ Women: over seven drinks per week, or three per occasion

- ♥ Men: over fourteen drinks per week, or four per occasion

Binge drinking

- ♥ Women: four or more drinks at one sitting

- ♥ Men: five or more drinks at one sitting

Much of the data available on alcohol and heart disease stems from research known as observational studies. While the information gleaned from such studies is OK, it is not as solid as data obtained from randomized trials or other more scientific methods. A primary problem with observational studies is relying on self-reported information. Whether intentionally or unintentionally, people are notoriously inaccurate in estimating how much they eat or drink. Observational studies are also subject to circumstantial biases. For example, people who have a glass of wine with dinner may also be more likely to eat heart-healthy foods, maintain their weight, exercise regularly, and avoid cigarettes. Teasing out which variable is protecting the heart—wine or other lifestyle choices—becomes a challenge.

Despite the plethora of observational data, there is still good information from other sources: prospective trials, cohort studies, survey analyses, and meta-analyses. All show a benefit in light or moderate alcohol consumption. In one such study moderate drinking reduced the risk for coronary heart disease by 40 to 70 percent—compared to heavy drinking or no drinking.[8]

Researchers have discovered this protective effect in all groups, including those who already have coronary heart disease, those without any heart disease, those with preexisting risk factors like diabetes, and the elderly. Not only does moderate drinking reduce the risk for a heart attack, but it also reduces the risk of death from a cardiac-related cause. The benefit applies to all beverages, although the association is stronger for wine than beer and liquor. The type of alcohol is not as important as the quantity and pattern of drinking.

There are several mechanisms that likely contribute to alcohol's protective effects against heart disease. For starters, HDL cholesterol increases by up to 10 percent among moderate drinkers.[9] Moderate amounts of alcohol may serve as an antioxidant, particularly substances like the flavonoids and phenolic compounds found in red wine. Human and animal studies also confirm that moderate drinking enhances the body's sensitivity to insulin, reduces the tendency for the body to form blood clots, and reduces inflammation. All of these factors relate to coronary events.

The key word is *moderate*. Across the board, researchers have learned the benefits of alcohol only come through light or moderate consumption. Heavy drinking and binge drinking are not beneficial to the heart. Interestingly, both heavy drinking and binge drinking are strong indicators of a loss of self-control. When we forsake God's favor by rejecting the fruit of the Spirit, we can expect an unfavorable outcome. On that note, I will conclude by examining the potential risks of alcohol.

Potential harm

Wine is a mocker and beer a brawler; whoever is led astray by them is not wise.

—Proverbs 20:1, niv

As we have seen, if we maintain control, alcohol can be beneficial. However, if we lose control, alcohol becomes a serious problem. Self-control governs whether we should drink at all (remember the issue of liberty), and it governs the way we drink—how much and how often. Once again the Bible affirms the dangers of unrestrained use:

♥ Proverbs 23:29–35 describes hazards that stem from uncontrolled drinking. Among potential consequences are sorrow, strife, injuries, cognitive impairment, and visual hallucinations.

♥ The apostle Peter uses drunkenness in discussing the unredeemed life. He tells believers this is the sort of lifestyle that should be part of their past, not their present: "For the time already past is sufficient for you to have carried out the desire of the Gentiles, having pursued a course of sensuality, lusts, drunkenness, carousals, drinking parties and abominable idolatries" (1 Peter 4:3, nas).

♥ An earlier passage in Proverbs 23 advises us to avoid even associating with heavy drinkers: "Do not be with heavy drinkers of wine, or with gluttonous eaters of meat; for the heavy drinker and the glutton will come to poverty" (Proverbs 23:20–21, nas).

Alcohol's potential for destruction goes beyond physical health: injuries, accidents, impaired job performance, and strained relationships. Then there are its general health consequences, such as liver damage, brain damage, and various cancers, including breast cancer. In addition, alcohol can specifically damage the heart, both through cardiovascular disease and other ways.

Binge drinking increases the risk for heart attack. One meta-analysis (which gathers information from several studies and reaches conclusions based on these pooled results) found that the relative risk for both fatal and nonfatal heart attacks increased among binge drinkers, compared to those who did not drink heavily. Researchers defined binge drinking as consuming five or more drinks per occasion, or getting intoxicated at least once per month.[10]

Hypertension is a major risk factor for cardiovascular disease; excessive alcohol has a tendency to elevate blood pressure. Those who consume more than two drinks per day have up to a two-fold increase in the incidence of hypertension, compared to non-drinkers. This risk increases in proportion to the amount of alcohol consumed, with an especially high risk among people who consume more than five drinks per day.[11]

While light to moderate alcohol use may protect against the development of heart failure, excessive drinking can damage the heart muscles to the point of causing heart failure. This condition is known as "alcoholic cardiomyopathy." Heavy drinking and binge drinking can also cause atrial fibrillation, where the heart does not contract appropriately, causing an irregular heartbeat. Light to moderate drinking does not have this effect. Alcohol-induced heart failure and alcohol-related atrial fibrillation are not the consequences of coronary artery disease per se. Yet they demonstrate how excessive alcohol is toxic to the heart, in ways other than circulation problems.

Recommendations

> A simple man believes anything, but a prudent man gives thought to his steps.
>
> —Proverbs 14:15, NIV

Because alcohol use carries risks and benefits, I always strongly advise caution with its use. In many instances the risks heavily outweigh the benefits. In addition, as I mentioned previously, the data on alcohol come primarily from observational studies, which have their limitations. There are no large, long-term randomized and controlled trials to glean more precise information on the matter. For this reason I do not recommend alcohol as a means of lowering the risk for coronary artery disease. Other approaches to lifestyle modification, such as diet, exercise, and maintaining a healthy body weight, are better and safer ways to lower your risk.

The bottom line: If you don't drink, don't start. There are other ways to protect your heart. If you do drink, keep it light to moderate. If drinking is a problem, get some help to overcome it. Then permanently abstain from alcohol.

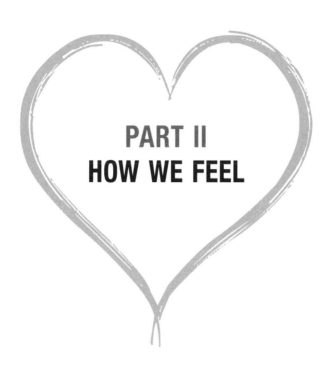

PART II
HOW WE FEEL

Chapter 4

CHOOSE A "HAPPY HEART"

A merry heart does good, like medicine,
but a broken spirit dries the bones.

Proverbs 17:22

EVERY OCCUPATION HAS ITS TOOLS OF THE TRADE: A HAMMER for the carpenter, a calculator for the accountant, and pills for the health care provider. After all, where would I be without my prescription pad (or, more accurately, electronic transmittal)? That said, some medical problems are best handled surgically and others best managed through a counselor's listening ear. For some ailments physical therapy is ideal. For others, the best remedy is avoiding whatever triggered the condition. And I will never forget the wise instruction of the medical school professor who taught us when to use the "tincture of time." In other words, patiently allow the body to heal itself.

While there are a wide variety of treatment options, medications—tablets, capsules, or elixirs—remain a valuable tool for the health care professional. Yet since no tool is perfect, one of the most troubling challenges of prescription medications is possible side effects. The potential for a medication to cause an adverse reaction can be quite serious—at times, enough for the drug's maker to pull it from the market. Thankfully most instances are few and far between; doctors, nurses, and pharmacists work together to minimize prescription-drug-related complications. Still they remain quite real. Just listen to the final segment of prescription drug commercials, when the announcer spits out a litany of potential complications. When the list includes "death" along with insomnia, constipation, hair loss, or skin rash, one can't help feeling concerned.

Another problem with our tools is that many are prohibitively expensive. Depending on the condition, the cost can run hundreds or thousands of dollars a month. Even with good health insurance providing prescription benefits, co-payments can prove rather pricey. For those on fixed incomes or little income, spending money on medications may not rank high on the priority list. When the choice comes down to eating or buying pills, you have the real-life definition of "squeezed."

A third barrier to using these tools effectively is the serious problem of health illiteracy. In health matters this goes beyond reading ability. It includes the ability to interpret, analyze, and evaluate health information; to clearly articulate health concerns; and to understand medical advice and directions for treatment. According to the Institute of Medicine, 90 million people (nearly half of all American adults) have difficulty comprehending and acting on health information.[1] As a result, mishaps are common. Such direction as which pill to take, how many times a day, and such specific directions as "take on an empty stomach" are often misunderstood.

We can't overlook another major barrier, which is the fact that many people simply don't want our tools. When I suggest a particular prescription, I often encounter apprehension, resistance, and even refusal. When the latter occurs, the patient-doctor relationship can deteriorate into a battle of wills. I hate it when that happens. It doesn't help to realize that many people who are horror-struck at the thought of taking a prescription drug (even one tiny little pill) are quite willing—even happy—to swallow a dozen or more dietary supplements they purchased online. Although few know what they are getting or its impact on their health, they believe a website or a friend's recommendation (taking "self-medication" to a new level).

The Free Prescription

So while we have a vast array of tools, success doesn't come easily. To the contrary, they include a host of challenges. However, it is nice to know a free medication exists that features no side effects and is never a source of confusion. That prescription is for a "merry heart," which according to Proverbs 17:22 works just like medicine. I am pleased to testify how well this tool works. I can heartily recommend it to everyone.

What exactly is a merry heart? First, you need to understand this term. Webster's Dictionary says *merry* means to be full of gaiety and high spirits, to be festive and jovial. The connotations (at least in our language) carry a hint of conditional happiness, though. In other words, I can be merry when my circumstances make me merry. However, if they change, my state of merriment might suffer a setback. However, this is not the essence of the word used in Proverbs. The Hebrew word is *sameach*, which means *bless* or *blessed*. So a merry heart is a blessed heart. *Blessed* literally means happy, fortunate, and blissful. It is the same word Jesus used repeatedly in the Beatitudes in the fifth chapter of Matthew:

> Blessed are the poor in spirit,
> For theirs is the kingdom of heaven.
> Blessed are those who mourn,
> For they shall be comforted.
> Blessed are the meek,
> For they shall inherit the earth.
> Blessed are those who hunger and thirst for righteousness,
> For they shall be filled.
> Blessed are the merciful,
> For they shall obtain mercy.

Blessed are the pure in heart,
For they shall see God.
Blessed are the peacemakers,
For they shall be called sons of God.
Blessed are those who are persecuted for righteousness' sake,
For theirs is the kingdom of heaven.

Blessed are you when they revile and persecute you, and say
all kinds of evil against you falsely for My sake. Rejoice and
be exceedingly glad, for great is your reward in heaven, for so
they persecuted the prophets who were before you.
—MATTHEW 5:3–12

Jesus listed these nine descriptions of *sameach* at the start of His Sermon on the Mount. None sound especially festive. This is because the state of blessedness is not contingent on our circumstances, nor is it governed by our emotions. It refers to a status God divinely grants to those who are faithful. We choose faithfulness, and in return God makes our hearts merry. So if a merry heart is like a medicine, how do we go about getting this prescription filled? Let's examine a few more proverbs to learn how.

Proverbs 3:13 says, "Happy is the man who finds wisdom, and the man who gains understanding." This verse speaks of divine wisdom. Rest assured, not all wisdom is divine. James describes two types of wisdom and makes a careful distinction between that which comes from God and the other, which originates with human reasoning. The wisdom from God is "first pure, then peaceable, gentle, willing to yield, full of mercy and good fruits, without partiality and without hypocrisy" (James 3:17). This is the wisdom Solomon repeatedly encourages us to embrace in the fourth chapter of Proverbs: the wisdom personified by God. Even Paul refers to Christ as "wisdom from God" (1 Corinthians 1:30). As we pursue divine wisdom, where we strengthen our relationship with God and yield to His precepts, we will reap the benefits of a happy heart.

Proverbs also tells us that being happy, or blessed, depends on how we treat others: "He who has mercy on the poor, happy is he" (Proverbs 14:21). This biblical happiness is diametrically opposed to happiness as defined by worldly values, which emphasize pleasing self. Supposedly taking a trendy vacation, wearing nice clothes, buying a new car, or acquiring an upscale home will lead to happiness. Yet it doesn't take long to learn that this form of "happiness" is neither enduring nor satisfying. True happiness comes from taking on the attributes of Christ, who "made himself nothing, taking the very nature of a servant" (Philippians 2:7, NIV). In doing so, He showed us mercy. When we strive to be more like Jesus, we treat others the way He treated us. We show kindness, compassion, and generosity, and place others' needs above our own. This is how we fill the prescription for a merry heart.

According to Proverbs, a merry heart trusts God: "Whoever trusts in the LORD, happy is he" (Proverbs 16:20). The kingdom of God has no place for worry. As Jesus said, "Therefore I say to you, do not worry about your life, what you will eat or what you will drink; nor about your body, what you will put on. Is not life more than food and the body more than clothing?" (Matthew 6:25). Paul advised, "Be anxious for nothing, but in everything by prayer and supplication, with thanksgiving, let your requests be made known to God" (Philippians 4:6). If a merry heart is like a medicine, then one way to void this divine prescription is through worry.

Indeed, a merry heart is therapeutic. Growing in wisdom, showing mercy, and learning to trust God rather than worrying will lead to blessings. We have a prescription for a tried and true medication with no co-payment or side effects. When we comply with the orders of Jesus—the Great Physician—we will reap the rewards He promised.

Optimism vs. Pessimism

All the days of the afflicted are evil, but he who is of a merry heart has a continual feast.

—PROVERBS 15:15

"Attitude is everything." For centuries this concept has been conveyed through speakers, writers, and folks who are just plain smart. Here are a few pearls of wisdom:

The only disability in life is a bad attitude.[2]

—SCOTT HAMILTON

Things turn out best for the people who make the best out of the way things turn out.[3]

—ART LINKLETTER

A happy person is not a person in a certain set of circumstances, but rather a person with a certain set of attitudes.[4]

—HUGH DOWNS

He who has so little knowledge of human nature as to seek happiness by changing anything but his own disposition will waste his life in fruitless efforts.[5]

—SAMUEL JOHNSON

Since the house is on fire let us warm ourselves.[6]

—ITALIAN PROVERB

Attitude makes a world of difference. Many of you have heard this or similar statements in books, lectures, and inspirational messages, to the point it may sound like a cliché. Yet it isn't. If more people "got it," there wouldn't be such a huge market for motivational speakers and self-help books. Since attitude is a choice, each person reading these words has access to the advantages that come from maintaining a positive disposition. Unlike our circumstances, which are often beyond our control, our attitude is a decision of the will. Embracing a positive outlook is one of the most powerful weapons at our disposal since it converts life's lemons into lemonade.

The tendency toward optimism or pessimism is described in one of two ways. Most people have what I refer to as either "dispositional optimism" or "dispositional pessimism." This is the tendency to embrace either a positive or negative outlook on life, whether about present circumstances or the future. Then there is the "explanatory" variety that explains life's events with either a positive or negative slant. Tools such as the Minnesota Multiphasic Personality Inventory (MMPI) can objectively measure a person's tendency toward optimism or pessimism. Through tools like the MMPI researchers have discovered the impact of attitude on physical well-being and quality of life.

When considering the benefits of a positive attitude, we can limit ourselves to psychosocial or emotional well-being. However, an upbeat disposition is beneficial to physical health too. One study found that two years after knee replacement surgery, pessimistic people had significantly more moderate to severe knee pain and less improvement in knee function, compared to optimistic people.[7] In addition, pessimists who suffer from chronic pain, who tend to focus their minds on their pain, and who feel helpless about the prospect of relief have higher levels of interleukin-6 in their bloodstream. (Interleukin-6 is a reliable indicator of chronic inflammation and may actually increase sensitivity to pain.)[8]

A pessimistic disposition can also negatively impact longevity. Researchers at the Mayo Clinic followed more than seven thousand people who completed the MMPI in the early 1960s. Over the next forty years they learned that people with pessimistic, anxious, and depressive personality traits had a higher rate of death, no matter what the cause.[9] A different study examined whether the way people explained life events had an impact on longevity. Over the course of thirty years, researchers followed more than seven hundred patients who had completed the MMPI. Researchers discovered that those with a more pessimistic style of interpretation had a 19 percent increased risk of mortality.[10]

Another study involving approximately five hundred elderly men and women showed similar results. In this study researchers classified the participants as having a "positive life orientation" if they answered "yes" to the following questions:

♥ Are you satisfied with life?

♥ Do you have zest for life?

♥ Do you have plans for the future?

♥ Do you feel needed?

♥ Do you seldom feel lonely or depressed?

After a decade, of the 20 percent of participants with a positive life orientation, 54.5 percent were still alive. That compared to 39.5 percent of those with a less-than-positive orientation. In addition, a positive attitude protected these individuals against the need for institutional care. After five years only 2.9 percent of positive responders were permanent residents of nursing homes or other institutions, compared to 17.5 percent of the rest.[11]

Positive Impact on Heart Health

A positive or negative attitude has a strong influence on heart health. In scores of studies examining the impact, the results are impressive. In these pages I cannot cite all the research that identifies a connection between a pessimistic disposition and coronary events such as angina or myocardial infarction—the data is far too extensive, and scientific investigation is active in this particular area. However, let's review a couple of them, starting with the landmark Women's Health Initiative (WHI).

Launched in 1991, this major project examined disease and causes of death among nearly 162,000 females from across the country, ages fifty to seventy-nine at the time of enrollment. The WHI represented a diverse sample of races, ethnicities, and socio-economic status. Investigators tracked them for more than fifteen years and gleaned a wealth of insights on postmenopausal hormone therapy, nutrition, osteoporosis, breast cancer, and—for our purposes—cardiovascular disease. At the start of the study each participant completed a questionnaire that assessed many variables, including optimism and pessimism. Researchers found that optimistic women had lower rates of coronary heart disease and lower rates of death from all causes; the most pessimistic had higher rates for both outcomes.[12]

In another study, researchers from Columbia University specifically examined the issue of positive vs. negative outlooks by using a five-point scale to quantify attitudes. They administered their scale to 1,700 men and women participating in the Canadian Nova Scotia Health Survey and followed them for ten years. During this time 145 suffered a heart attack. The researchers found that for every point scored on the five-point positivity scale, the participant's risk for a heart attack decreased by 20 percent.[13]

Not only is there a connection between pessimism and experiencing a coronary event, but also the Columbia researchers found that pessimism will also hinder and prolong recovery after an event. Optimistic people had a faster rate of recuperation after coronary artery bypass surgery and returned to normal activities sooner than pessimists. They also had a better quality of life six months after their operations.[14]

A different study of just over three hundred men and women who had coronary bypass surgery examined how often they needed readmittance to the hospital after discharge. Compared to optimistic people, pessimists were more likely to be rehospitalized for such reasons as wound infections, myocardial infarction, angina, or the need to undergo a second bypass.[15] This connection applies to other parts of the cardiovascular system. Compared to pessimistic people, optimists have:

♥ Fewer strokes[16]

♥ A slower progression of carotid artery disease[17]

The connection between optimism and heart health is clear—your outlook will have an impact on heart health. The next question, then, is: What can you do about it? Anyone who has lived with a negative person (or if you *are* that person) will attest to the difficulty of changing someone's disposition. As we grow older, a "bah-humbug" nature can become so ingrained that change seems virtually impossible. Nevertheless, we have a tool at our disposal that has the capacity to transform our nature and instill hope in even a lifelong Scrooge. That tool is gratitude. For the sake of our hearts, we must learn to be thankful.

The Power of Gratitude

> In everything give thanks; for this is the will of God in Christ Jesus for you.
> —1 THESSALONIANS 5:18

Paul closed his first letter to the church in Thessalonica with a series of directives, including this verse. When studying the Bible, it helps to keep the historical setting in mind even though it applies to all of us today. At the time Paul wrote this epistle, the church was experiencing intense persecution. Those who professed Jesus Christ as Savior and Lord faced personal attacks—some life-threatening. Yet Paul admonished them to be thankful. He even elaborated on the "when" and "why": we should be thankful "in everything." The reason: because "this is the will of God."

In my opinion, this verse is profound because it is so diametrically opposed to our natural inclinations. If left to the natural mind, the *time* to be thankful would be when great things happen to us, and the *reason* because great things take place. To the ordinary human mind gratitude is conditional. However, this ought not to be the case for Christ's followers. Much like the attribute of love, thankfulness should be ingrained in our character. This quality will set us apart from the world, enabling us to be grateful no matter what the circumstances.

Not only is gratitude God's will for us, but it also provides the best defense against pessimism. The two are like oil and water— they just don't mix. Pessimism brings with it the dark qualities of cynicism, distrust, and gloom. Thankfulness is like a light, able to drive out darkness and replace it with gladness, hopefulness, and confidence.

The Bible illustrates an example of the consequences of ingratitude in Exodus, when the Israelites found themselves in the wilderness after their miraculous delivery from Egypt.

Many of us know the story, albeit some from the long-running 1956 film *The Ten Commandments*, which starred Charlton Heston and Yul Brynner. Or from DreamWorks' 1998 animation *The Prince of Egypt*. Israel's exodus marked the end of a four-hundred-year period of severe oppression and slavery in Egypt. Certainly the family of Joseph—his father, brothers, wives, and children— were not perfect when they relocated to Egypt. Still, it seems institutional slavery planted seeds of negativity in their descendants, which took root and bore fruit over four hundred years. This is not surprising, especially since they were keenly aware of their status as God's chosen people. Enslavement must have been all the more painful in light of God's promises to Abraham. Their covenant of hope didn't include slavery, and "hope deferred makes the heart sick" (Proverbs 13:12).

God called on the Hebrew man named Moses to deliver his pessimistic brethren. Though Jewish by birth, Moses grew up in Egyptian culture, making him ideally suited to engage the powerful pharaoh who ruled the nation. And, despite his roots, Moses had never experienced the oppression of slavery, which must have spared him from the pessimism we see in the majority of his people.

The Hebrews displayed both types of pessimism—dispositional and explanatory.

First, they had a negative outlook on life (present and future) and were chronic complainers. Nothing was right, nothing was good, and nothing met their satisfaction, which meant they peppered their conversation with gripes—so much so that this constant grumbling made them irrational. At one point their dissatisfaction with manna led them to reflect nostalgically on their past life: "Who will give us meat to eat? We remember the fish which we ate freely in Egypt, the cucumbers, the melons, the leeks, the onions, and the garlic; but now our whole being is dried up; there is nothing at all except this manna before our eyes!" (Numbers 11:4–6). Somehow they forgot that in Egypt they endured centuries of oppression and tasty food brought with it a lack of freedom. This same kind of outlook can still make you illogical.

They were also explanatory pessimists, explaining life's events in a negative fashion. Consider the Israelites' gripes when they grew thirsty: "Then all the congregation of the children of Israel set out on their journey from the Wilderness of Sin, according to the commandment of the Lord, and camped in Rephidim; but there was no water for the people to drink. Therefore the people contended with Moses, and said, 'Give us water, that we may drink.' And Moses said to them, 'Why do you contend with me? Why do you tempt the Lord?' And the people thirsted there for water, and the people complained against Moses, and said, 'Why is it you have brought us up out of Egypt, to kill us and our children and our livestock with thirst?'" (Exodus 17:1–3).

Considering their location and desert climate, a water shortage shouldn't have surprised them. Yet the negative way the Israelites interpreted conditions revealed their nature. In their minds, a lack of water did not grant them another opportunity to see God perform a miracle. They did not view thirst as a means to strengthen their faith, nor did they see it as an occasion to learn a valuable lesson in endurance. Instead they resorted to blaming Moses, even wildly accusing him of hatching a conspiracy to kill them.

Pessimists in every sense of the word, they reached this outlook by choice. Although years of slavery and oppression may have planted and nurtured this disposition, they had the capacity to change. All they had to do was choose an attitude of gratitude. The root of their problem lay in thanklessness. Although they occasionally showed gratitude, it was conditional. This is the same as ingratitude, if not worse. For example, they threw a big praise party after crossing the Red Sea and witnessing the destruction of Pharaoh's army. As soon as difficulties appeared, though, their appreciation vanished. They did not give thanks "in everything" but only in those things that met with their satisfaction. Instead of following God's will, they allowed pessimism to govern them.

The evidence comes from their constant complaining, tendency to cast blame, and what I call a "wicked amnesia." When confronted by trials in the wilderness they forgot how much God loved them and the miraculous ways in which He had delivered them. If they had just remembered God's mercy and kindness when facing tribulation, optimism would have replaced pessimism. Likewise, when we reflect on past victories, we are better equipped to endure present trials and embrace hope for the future. In the biblical account after the wilderness experience, God regularly reminded Israel how He delivered them from Egypt and into the Promised Land; Psalms 105 and 106 recalls these events. I find it interesting that the early part of both psalms includes the decree: "Oh, give thanks to the LORD!" Reflecting on what God has done is indeed a safeguard against ingratitude.

We know that except for Joshua and Caleb, all of the Israelites above the age of twenty who came out of Egypt died in the wilderness and never saw the Promised Land. The fire of God's wrath consumed some (Numbers 11:1; 16:35); others were swallowed by the earth for their rebellion (Numbers 16:28–34). Some were executed for disobedience by their brother's sword (Exodus 32:25–28) and others bitten by fiery serpents for speaking against Moses and God (Numbers 21:4–6). What the Bible doesn't reveal is whether many suffered from cardiovascular disease. No doubt many would have died long before they had aged enough to develop significant atherosclerosis.

The point here is that had they chosen to be thankful in all things, instead of ungrateful in everything, their pessimistic outlook and tendency to rebel would have faded. This would have spared them from forty years of aimless wandering in the desert. They could have avoided death from any of the causes I mentioned in the previous paragraph. Most importantly, they could have entered the Promised Land with happy hearts. The root of their pessimism stemmed from thanklessness, which expressed itself in rebellion. This sealed their doom and caused premature death. Likewise, a negative disposition can still lead to an early demise. Learn the power of gratitude, and let thanksgiving preserve your heart.

Chapter 5

STRESS AND ANXIETY

Let not your heart be troubled...

John 14:1, KJV

N O MATTER WHAT OUR AGE, WE WILL CONFRONT SITUA-
tions with the potential to cause stress and anxiety, whether
individual incidents or chronic conditions. Jesus told His disciples, "In this world you will have trouble" (John 16:33, NIV). In his
description of the nature of trials, James used "when" rather than
"if": "Consider it all joy, my brethren, *when* you encounter various
trials" (James 1:2, NAS, emphasis added). Peter advised, "In this
you greatly rejoice, though now for a little while, if need be, you
have been grieved by various trials." (1 Peter 1:6). In other words,
trials are coming. It is just a matter of when they arrive and how
we respond.

The promise of tribulation applies to everyone—a kind of across-
the-board guarantee for any individual or group. So the question is:
How do we handle it? Or, more appropriately: What is the *biblical*
way to cope? While there are *unbiblical* ways to deal with adversity,
they are often detrimental. We must learn to cope in the way Christ
described in the latter part of John 16:33 "But take heart! I have
overcome the world" (NIV). We must also follow James's advice and
confront hard times with joy; when we do, we will reap the benefits
he promises in James 1:3 that "the testing of your faith produces

endurance" (NAS). Likewise, Peter says that when we withstand our trials, the genuineness of our faith will be "more precious than gold that perishes, though it is tested by fire [and] found to praise, honor, and glory at the revelation of Jesus Christ" (1 Peter 1:7).

The Bible regularly instructs us to guard against anxiety. Paul told us to "be anxious for nothing" (Philippians 4:6) while Jesus counseled, "Therefore I tell you, do not worry about your life, what you will eat or drink; or about your body, what you will wear" (Matthew 6:25, NIV). The verse that I opened this chapter with comes from a section in the Gospel of John where Jesus spoke to His disciples at His last meal with them. Since Judas Iscariot had already left the group, those remaining were true believers.

Jesus shared many things in the hours before His arrest and crucifixion, including the fact that His physical presence with them was drawing to a close. Being omniscient, Jesus knew of coming events and the feelings they would stir among the disciples. A myriad of negative emotions would threaten them: fear, disappointment, depression, anger, doubt, and feelings of abandonment and rejection. So, although Christ was about to face the greatest trial of all time, He chose to offer the disciples words of wisdom and comfort.

After telling them *not* to be anxious, He immediately explained *why* they had no reason to be anxious: "In My Father's house are many mansions; if it were not so, I would have told you. I go to prepare a place for you" (John 14:2). Because we have eternal hope, anxiety has no place in the heart of a believer. The world's trials and tribulations are temporary. Whatever happens in the "here and now" has no bearing on our eternity. If life itself is fleeting, so are its troubles.

Not only do we have hope for eternity, but we also have the assurance of our Father's sovereignty. We can take comfort in knowing that nothing will confront us without first passing through His loving hands. He is in total control of our lives and has authority over our circumstances. We can rest on the promise that God "will not let you be tempted beyond what you can bear" (1 Corinthians

10:13, NIV) and that "in all things God works for the good of those who love him, who have been called according to his purpose" (Romans 8:28, NIV).

Prone to Anxiety

Despite our knowledge of God's assurance, and even when we make a personal commitment to stand firm on the Bible's promises, humans are still prone to anxiety. Anxiety disorders affect about 18 percent of the US population, or approximately 40 million people.[1] They come in many forms, such as generalized anxiety disorders, obsessive-compulsive disorders, panic disorders, and various phobias. Although the connection between psychiatric disorders and cardiovascular disease is fairly established with respect to depression, there is not nearly as much evidence linking heart disease with anxiety disorders. This does not mean one does not exist. Intuitively we are aware of a connection. Because of a lack of medical studies confirming this association, we don't yet have "black and white" evidence needed to draw conclusions and guide therapy.

However, in recent years, researchers have taken a closer look at anxiety disorders and cardiovascular disease. For example, the Heart and Soul Study evaluated more than one thousand patients with coronary heart disease. It found that participants with a generalized anxiety disorder had a 62 percent higher rate of a recurrent event (heart attack, heart failure, or stroke) or death from cardiovascular disease than those who had a more relaxed outlook.[2]

As our knowledge grows through such studies, we will have a greater understanding of how to address problems scientifically. Thankfully we already have insights on addressing them spiritually, such as by keeping the right perspective. While life's day-to-day challenges can appear immense, in the wider view they are quite small. We tend to focus on smaller things—life's daily stressors—and forget the bigger picture. Remember, our eternity is secure.

God, who loves us, is in total control. The key to reducing anxiety is to habitually look at day-to-day events against the backdrop of eternity. Anxiety is reliable evidence that we have lost perspective. Worry occurs when we focus on relatively small circumstances and forget about God's love, sovereignty, and the eternal security He promised us (remember those "many mansions" Jesus described).

Paul spoke to the importance of keeping the right perspective: "Finally, brethren, whatever things are true, whatever things are noble, whatever things are just, whatever things are pure, whatever things are lovely, whatever things are of good report, if there is any virtue and if there is anything praiseworthy; meditate on these things" (Philippians 4:8). Troubling times serve a great purpose by teaching us, imparting wisdom, and pushing us toward maturity in such areas as patience and endurance. They also equip us to help others. However, one thing they do not accomplish is teaching us to govern our souls. When we allow it, adversity—which has the potential to bless us—becomes a curse that can devastate our minds and destroy our bodies.

The Physical Impact of Emotions

I will walk within my house with a perfect heart.
—PSALM 101:2, KJV

While life's difficult situations are tangible, their impact on our bodies starts within a less tangible place—our minds. Thoughts are not concrete; we cannot harness the things that preoccupy us and examine them in a test tube. Still, in this realm we analyze and process the events of life. Our minds activate our emotions, whose effects on our bodies are quite real. From a physiologic standpoint, what occurs mentally has measurable outcomes physically. Our emotions cause changes in the concentration of various substances, like hormones and steroids that circulate in our bloodstream.

Emotions influence the amount of resistance and turbulence within our blood vessels. They affect our organs—including the heart—in ways that are anything but intangible.

These effects are helpful under certain circumstances. When confronted with adversity, our bodies respond rapidly with a surge of "fight-or-flight" activity. They release helpful chemicals and stimulate other changes that equip us to either run away from the threat or stand and fight. The capacity to respond to danger can potentially save our lives, but what if the situation is not life-threatening or not even dangerous? If we forsake biblical precepts and "let our hearts be troubled" and are "anxious for everything," the body still releases those chemicals and causes physiologic changes. Instead of being advantageous to our survival, though, they become detrimental. Let me share a personal example.

A native Chicagoan, I live just outside the city. Chicago has a history of serious snowstorms. As I write this chapter, the impact of the blizzard of 2011 (third largest in history) is still fresh in my mind. It reminded me of 1999, when I worked in the city and drove to the office every day. (Chicago is also known for its grueling commutes.) On the day of the '99 storm, I didn't heed weather and traffic reports, so I didn't leave my office any earlier than normal. By the time I got into my car, travel times had escalated in inverse proportion to slowing traffic. Not surprisingly, the interstate was clogged. Halfway home, traffic had crawled to a standstill.

There I sat, along with what looked like thousands of other commuters. As minutes turned into hours, I fidgeted and developed painful tension in my head, neck, and shoulder muscles. As the first hour crept into the second, I grew preoccupied with anxious thoughts: What if I run out of gas? What if I have to use the bathroom? What if the snowplows can't get through? My breathing turned rapid and shallow. By the third hour, I neared total panic. When I arrived home five hours after leaving my office, I felt like a ball of nerves. I had subjected my body to several hours of a "fight-or-flight" response when there was no place to go, nobody to fight, and nothing to run away from.

I lost any sense of tranquility because I didn't allow my mind to think about the things of God, instead directing my attention onto my circumstances. Reflecting on this later, I realized how this seemingly terrible trouble was as permanent as a snowman on a sunny day. Hypothetically, what if we travelers were forsaken by our families and forgotten by the Chicago Department of Streets and Sanitation? What if the snowplows, salt trucks, and tow trucks had decided to leave us stranded? That would surely be the worst case scenario, but even then our trial would have been temporary. Snow is destined to melt eventually. So even amid the worst possible outcome of complete abandonment, I would still have been all right. I had subjected myself to physiologic harm—and all for naught.

What, then, occurred inside my body to provoke the symptoms of a panic attack? Several things took place as a result of my acute anxiety; such changes occur to some degree under a variety of other social and psychological states. Some examples include depression, chronic life stress, and social isolation. Doctors have observed similar, physiologic changes in people with pessimistic, angry, and hostile personalities, and adults subjected to harsh conditions like abuse or neglect as a child. All can affect the heart. This is an area of ongoing research that will shed more light on the subject. Yet what we have learned to date is quite significant.

Just as physical factors like hypertension, dyslipidemia, diabetes, smoking, and aging play a major role in cardiovascular disease, so does psychosocial stress—regardless of race, culture, or ethnicity. This finding emerged from data gleaned in INTERHEART, a multinational study designed to examine coronary artery disease risk factors. It included more than twenty-five thousand participants from more than fifty nations. The psychosocial factors surveyed included depression, adverse life events, the sense of a loss of control, perceived stress at home or at work, and financial difficulties. The results showed a substantial cardiac risk attributable to psychosocial factors alone, comparable to such other traditional risk factors as hypertension and smoking.[3]

Wide-Ranging Impact

The physiologic impact of stress is wide-ranging. For our purposes I will review the effects on the cardiovascular system in four categories: endothelial cells, stress mediators, platelet function, and inflammation. Keep in mind that while our bodies are extremely complex, I will try to keep things simple. Remember too that none of these systems work in isolation; all interact one with another. For instance, stress mediators affect the endothelium, which influences the inflammatory response, which impacts platelet function—and so on. Let's break them down.

Endothelial cell dysfunction

Our blood vessels are made up of layers of different types of tissue. The innermost layer, which lines the lumen and comes in direct contact with the blood, is covered with cells known as endothelial cells. These adhere to blood vessel walls and to each other, forming a complex, highly active network called the endothelium. This network is so large the endothelium can be considered a separate organ. These cells are found in all blood vessels (arteries, veins, and capillaries) and their functioning is vital to good health. Endothelial cells regulate our circulation by releasing substances that either dilate or constrict the arteries, which controls the rate of blood flow. Endothelial cells send signals that trigger inflammation and clotting. If our arteries are diseased by atherosclerosis, or if we have risk factors for it (e.g., hypertension, diabetes, smoking, dyslipidemia, and aging), we are predisposed to endothelial cell dysfunction.

The endothelium is sensitive to psychosocial stress. Several studies conducted on animals and humans show that mental stress can lead to endothelium-mediated constriction of the coronary arteries. This can compromise blood circulation to the heart. Even brief periods of mental stress, similar to what occurs in everyday life, can cause transient problems within endothelial cells that can last for up to four hours. This happens in people with preexisting atherosclerosis, but it also occurs in young, healthy people with no risk factors for coronary artery disease.[4]

As I mentioned, the endothelium also controls the formation and propagation of blood clots, an extremely important function with respect to heart attack and stroke.

Stress mediators

Several substances in the body—hormones, steroids, and other chemicals—can be collectively referred to as "stress mediators." Some are controlled by a part of the brain known as the hypothalamus. It sends signals to the pituitary and adrenal glands that either stimulate or suppress the release of a variety of chemicals, including cortisol (a steroid) and various growth and sex hormones. Other stress mediators are made by the body's nerves, with the most significant contribution coming from the sympathetic nervous system. This system releases chemicals called catecholamines. Norepinephrine and epinephrine are both catecholamines and play a major role in the body's "fight-or-flight" response.

Activation of the sympathetic nervous system affects many parts of the body, including the cardiovascular system—heart rate increases, heart contractions become stronger, and blood pressure rises. As previously mentioned, in the face of danger the ability to respond in this way can preserve our life. However, depending on the intensity of the response, if the coronary arteries are diseased from atherosclerosis or the heart muscle is abnormal, the heart may not be able to withstand heightened stimulation. In addition, catecholamines released by the sympathetic nervous system have the capacity to disrupt regular heartbeat. This can trigger fatal heart rhythms, such as ventricular fibrillation. When the body releases stress mediators in response to psychological and social conditions, they have the same effect as when released in response to danger. In acute cases the heart may get overstimulated to the point of death.

There are also significant cardiovascular risks with the chronic secretion of stress mediators. Many people live with constant psychosocial stress, either from life's challenges, difficult relationships, mental illness, or a combination of these factors. These circumstances can subject the body to long-term effects of stress, impacting the heart directly and indirectly. For example, chronic secretion of cortisol is associated with central obesity. This means fat accumulates in and around internal organs inside our body cavity—instead of just beneath our skin. As I discussed previously, this type of fat distribution is a hallmark for insulin resistance and is a precursor to type 2 diabetes and cardiovascular disease. Cortisol plays a role in hypertension through increasing blood pressure. It also alters the lipids to a "heart-unfriendly" profile, with elevation in LDL-cholesterol and triglyceride levels and a decrease in HDL (good cholesterol). Diabetes, hypertension, and dyslipidemia are all major risk factors for heart disease.

Platelet function

Our blood is a heterogeneous substance made up of fluid, cells, proteins, and small particles called platelets. People with abnormal or deficient platelets, which are instrumental in blood clotting, have a tendency to bleed excessively. Platelets also play a major role in cardiovascular disease, which is why aspirin and other anti-platelet medications are so useful in the prevention of heart attacks.

When activated, platelets gather together and become sticky. This aggregate forms the core of a clot, called a "thrombus." In coronary artery disease, a thrombus helps clog the coronary blood vessel, causing unstable angina, myocardial infarction, or sudden cardiac death. Several things can trigger platelet activation. With respect to heart disease, endothelial damage caused by atherosclerosis tops this list. Coronary arteries diseased by atherosclerosis develop fat-laden rough spots known as "plaques." These plaques line the lumen of the blood vessels, which inhibits blood flow—hence the terms "clogged arteries" or "blocked arteries."

Some plaques are more prone to rupture than others. When they rupture, the endothelium releases substances to activate platelets and forms a thrombus, compromising circulation. Many things can precipitate plaque rupture and platelet activation. Although at this time the data is not entirely conclusive, some studies suggest that mental stress enhances platelet aggregation through activating the sympathetic nervous system.[5]

Inflammation

Our bodies feature an extremely complex system to protect us against infection and facilitate healing after an injury. The initial response leads to inflammation, a process that involves action by a wide variety of cells and the various chemicals they secrete. Like the release of stress mediators, inflammation can help preserve life under the proper circumstances. However, when it turns into a chronic condition, it becomes detrimental to health.

Determining the degree of inflammation comes by measuring the number of inflammatory cells, measuring the chemicals they secrete, and evaluating other changes. Collectively these are called "markers of inflammation." Both endothelial cells and platelets can trigger inflammation, which is part of a cascade of events that culminate in the formation of a thrombus. High levels of inflammatory markers are predictive of cardiovascular events in healthy men and women as well as in people with coronary artery disease.

Interestingly people with conditions that cause any type of inflammation have a greater predisposition to heart disease. For instance, rheumatoid arthritis and systemic lupus erythematosus (SLE) are collagen vascular diseases that cause chronic inflammation, especially in the joints. People diagnosed with these conditions, particularly women, have a significantly higher risk for myocardial infarction.[6] Poor oral hygiene with tooth decay and chronic periodontitis is also associated with increased risk for cardiovascular disease, with chronic inflammation being the likely culprit.[7]

While psychosocial stress can affect the endothelium, stress also modifies cells in the bloodstream—such as macrophages, which play a key role in inflammation.[8] In addition, chronic stress can trigger the production of inflammatory markers from other tissues throughout the body, including fat cells.

Aside from these physiologic effects, people subjected to chronic psychosocial stress are more likely to engage in behaviors that negatively impact the heart. The tendencies to smoke and to drink heavily will increase with escalating levels of stress. Some respond to adversity by overeating, which can lead to weight gain and attending consequences, including type 2 diabetes. To add insult to injury, excess cortisol stimulates our craving for sweet and fatty foods.[9] In other words, stress doesn't prompt people to reach for vegetables and whole grains, which would at least confer some health benefits. Instead, stressed overeaters tend to select highly processed, high-calorie foods and beverages with excessive amounts of saturated fat (causing dyslipidemia), salt (blood pressure problems) and added sugar (obesity).

This typical reaction to stress shows how it can destroy the motivation needed for proper self-care. Cooking nutritious meals and engaging in regular exercise will fall low on the priority list for people experiencing stress. Certainly all of these secondary consequences play a significant role in increasing the risk for heart disease. Let's now look at some specific data on the heart's response to acute and chronic stress.

Acute Stress

And they said to him, Joseph is still alive! And he is governor over all the land of Egypt! And Jacob's heart began to stop beating and [he almost] fainted, for he did not believe them.
—GENESIS 45:26, AMP

Long before the invention of the strange-sounding sphygmomanometer to measure blood pressure, long before we had laboratories with equipment to quantify the level of catecholamines in the circulation, long before there were cardiac monitors to accurately record the heart's rhythm, and long before we could visualize our insides using technology such as positron emission tomography and radionuclide ventriculography, we knew that something happened to the heart in response to acute stress.

The biblical account of Joseph includes a vivid description of Jacob's reaction when he learned that his favorite son was still alive. For decades Jacob had believed that Joseph died a violent death; initially this false report filled him with overwhelming grief. However, even the good news proved stressful, especially for an old man. Why? Quite possibly his sympathetic nervous system released a surge of catecholamines into his bloodstream. This could have triggered a transient arrhythmia, such as ventricular tachycardia or ventricular fibrillation. This is why his heart slowed down. Compromised blood circulation reduced the amount of oxygen delivered to his brain, causing him to faint. Or it is possible the news stimulated a critical nerve in his brain, slowing his heart rate significantly. In either case, although the effects proved temporary, this stress-inducing revelation impacted his heart in a potentially fatal way.

Acute stress can have adverse effects on the heart. A few large community-based studies have shown a strong association between stress and cardiac events—not only among people diagnosed with psychiatric conditions (panic disorder or generalized anxiety disorder) but the general population as well. One large study followed approximately 34,000 male health care professionals with no evidence of cardiovascular disease. Over a two-year period the risk of sudden cardiac death was significantly higher in men who tended to be anxious, compared to those who were not.[10] Interestingly, in these men excess risk only surfaced with sudden cardiac death; anxiety had no impact on the incidence of nonfatal myocardial infarction. This points toward the potential for stress to affect (among other things) the rhythm of the heart, since fatal arrhythmias like ventricular fibrillation precipitate sudden cardiac death.

Another group of investigators reviewed death certificates from Los Angeles County before and after the Northridge Earthquake on January 17, 1994. For the first sixteen days of January, authorities attributed an average of 73 deaths per day to cardiac causes. On the day of the earthquake, this number rose to 125, a clear indication of the impact of acute stress on the heart.[11]

Two other studies looked at how the terrorist attacks on the World Trade Center on September 11, 2001, affected people in New York and Florida, respectively. Both examined the records of men and women who had implantable cardioverter-defibrillators (ICDs), which are devices used in people with heart disease that help maintain a normal heart rhythm. Whenever the heart develops a potentially harmful rhythm, the device discharges a small electrical shock to restore a normal beating pattern. ICDs have the capacity to record and store this data for months. The first study found that after the New York attacks, the rate of ventricular arrhythmias increased by twofold.[12] The second found nearly identical results in ICD patients in Florida, even though the attack didn't occur within their geographic proximity.[13]

Catecholamines released by the sympathetic nervous system have the capacity to trigger arrhythmias. However, activation of the sympathetic nervous system also causes the heart rate, blood pressure, and the force of heart contractions to intensify. So even if the heart maintains a normal rhythm, this combination will increase the heart's need for oxygen—and the presence of coronary artery disease compromises oxygen delivery in several ways. This can include a constriction of blood vessels within the heart muscle (a consequence of catecholamine release), partial artery blockage by atherosclerosis plaques, or a complete blockage. In addition, the increase in heart rate and blood pressure can generate stress within blood vessels that can damage the endothelium. This can trigger inflammation, platelet activation, and clot formation.

So acute stress can precipitate arrhythmias, endothelial damage, and clot formation. Even though far less common, there is another stress-related heart disorder worth noting. First described in Japan, *takotsubo* is the Japanese word for "octopus trap." This disorder causes the tissue of the heart to dilate and become "floppy" (for lack of a better term), giving it a trap-like appearance. While not really an *artery* problem, it is related to dysfunction in the *muscles* of the heart. In the United States we call it stress-induced cardiomyopathy, apical ballooning syndrome, or—more commonly—broken heart syndrome.

This condition is much more common in older women. In one review of data from ten reports on the disorder, women generally between the ages of sixty-one and seventy-six made up between 80 and 100 percent of the cases.[14] It is usually triggered by intense emotional or physical stress; for example, the unexpected death of a loved one, devastating financial loss, domestic violence, or receiving catastrophic news such as diagnosis of a terminal illness. The symptoms mimic that of an acute myocardial infarction, with chest pain, shortness of breath, and abnormalities on an electrocardiogram. The coronary arteries, however, are usually entirely normal or have minimal atherosclerosis. Yet the ventricle of the heart—a normally firm muscle with strong, effective contractions—becomes dilated and slack, which diminishes its capacity to pump blood and maintain adequate blood pressure. The result: heart failure, shock, or a variety of arrhythmias.

Although we don't know the cause of stress-induced

cardiomyopathy with 100 percent certainty, it most likely stems from a surge of catecholamines released by the sympathetic nervous system in response to severe emotional or physical trauma. Although temporary, it can reoccur. In patients who survive the initial episode, the heart typically recovers functions over the course of one to four weeks. And while acute stress has a profound effect on the heart, chronic stress also impacts the heart—though not as dramatically, the consequences are still significant.

Chronic Stress

The churning inside me never stops; days of suffering confront me.
—JOB 30:27, NIV

While focusing on the effects of stress on the heart, I should note that it impacts many other parts of our bodies. Job's account gives examples of acute and chronic stress. The acute stress takes place in the first two chapters. Over the course of one day Job loses everything when one calamity after another strikes. It starts with his wealth (and he was quite wealthy) and follows with all his children. In chapter 2 Job loses his health and vitality, including Satan striking him with painful boils from head to toe. After a week— enough time for the initial surge of stress mediators to dissipate— Job discusses his situation with three friends. It is obvious Job is experiencing the physical manifestations of chronic stress; he calls it a "churning inside." This involves more than his heart; he feels anguish in every aspect of his being—physically, mentally and emotionally.

While not many people have experienced calamities that match what Job endured, life is still full of hardships. As with Job, many are unexpected. People from all walks of life experience turmoil and strain on many fronts, whether related to the economy, employment, relationships, or other factors. Such long-term stressors can certainly affect our health. Several variables contribute to chronic stress, including:

♥ Inadequate social support

♥ Low socioeconomic status

♥ Work stress

♥ Close relationships, including marriage

Social support refers to those people and systems linked to an individual, collectively referred to as a "social network." In the past several years our ability to contact people, whether through online, smartphone, or other high-tech means, has exploded. However, social support entails more than just the capacity to connect (which I will discuss in more detail in the next chapter).

The second factor, socioeconomic status, includes education, income, occupation, and social status, or a combination of these. For nearly a century research has identified an inverse relationship between socioeconomic status and death. A low socioeconomic status confers a higher rate of mortality, and vice versa. This association exists for all causes of death, not just cardiovascular disease. Much excess mortality is a consequence of lifestyle—smoking, poor diet, and inadequate exercise are more common among people in low socioeconomic groups. Yet there is more to it than that.

While lifestyle plays a role, so does chronic stress generated by such elements as poor housing conditions, exposure to crime (particularly violent crime), and the financial hardships that often go hand in hand with low socioeconomic status. One consequence of such stress is that the body loses its ability to regulate cortisol (a steroid secreted by the adrenal gland in response to stress). The amount delivered into the bloodstream is regulated by an extremely complex, finely tuned system. However, when the body secretes excess cortisol, it throws off this precisely regulated system.

One study designed to examine the role of socioeconomic status and cortisol measured cortisol levels throughout the workday in nearly three hundred middle-aged men from various socioeconomic groups. They ranged from manual laborers to civil servants to university graduates. Researchers learned that manual laborers' bodies released larger amounts of cortisol in response to everyday stress and did not regulate cortisol levels normally. Compared to men in higher socioeconomic groups, they also had larger waist measurements, the result of cortisol-mediated abdominal fat accumulation.[15]

It is worth noting that stress from a low socioeconomic status tends to overlap with the third factor, work-related stress. However, not everyone experiencing work-related stress comes from a lower socioeconomic strata. Nor should work be pigeon-holed as the leading source of stress. While many misinterpret work as part of the "curse" that followed Adam and Eve's fall, the opportunity and ability to work is a blessing from God. It is also His expectation for mankind; before the Fall God employed Adam as a caretaker for the Garden of Eden (Genesis 2:15).

Ideally our work should be satisfying and fulfilling, but that is not always the case. Sometimes work can become a psychological burden that damages our health:

- ♥ Some jobs do not allow employees to use their intellect in making decisions or completing tasks. Workers can feel confined and restricted in terms of creativity.

- ♥ Other jobs are hectic, with great demands placed on employees—both physical and psychological.

In both circumstances the risk for coronary heart disease increases.[16]

Likewise, we can experience chronic stress when our work provides few rewards, such as career advancement, enhanced self-esteem, financial incentives, or job security. This "effort-reward" imbalance has also been linked to adverse cardiovascular events.[17]

That brings us to the fourth chronic stress factor, close

relationships. Research has linked marital stress to an increase in the risk of coronary heart disease in women. One group of investigators followed women who had an acute myocardial infarction or unstable angina approximately five years after initial hospitalization. During that interval women experiencing high stress in marriage or a cohabitating relationship had a nearly threefold greater risk of having another myocardial infarction or dying from cardiovascular disease.[18]

However, marital satisfaction has an opposite effect. In another study, investigators discovered high-quality marriages protected women against cardiovascular disease. They conducted surveys of marital status and satisfaction among nearly four hundred women. After more than a decade they evaluated participants for evidence of atherosclerosis. They found that the arteries of women in satisfying marriages had significantly less atherosclerotic plaque buildup and a less rapid progression of atherosclerosis, when compared to dissatisfied spouses. The degree of atherosclerosis in women who were single fell somewhere in between.[19]

The Wisdom of Christ

I opened this chapter with Jesus's admonition, "Let not your heart be troubled." In view of the scientific findings I have cited, Christ's words ought to take on added significance. And His advice applies in more ways than one. Life's challenges produce stress that affects the heart in a figurative sense. However, anxiety, fretfulness, and emotional fatigue can damage our hearts physically! The emotional "heart" and the four-chambered muscle within the chest cavity are both vulnerable to stress. Since Jesus promised that stressful events are part of life, I think it is appropriate to conclude with a brief overview of some approaches that can minimize the detrimental effects.

As a qualifier, for those who believe in Christ, a biblical approach to stress management should be a given. Prayer, meditation, and governing our thoughts are part of Christian living, regardless of life's trials. They become especially important if you have a predisposition toward anxiety. Through the Holy Spirit, God equipped us to "take captive every thought to make it obedient to Christ" (2 Corinthians 10:5, NIV). This includes thoughts that cause potentially detrimental physiologic changes—like those I experienced during that Chicago snowstorm.

For some Christians this approach is adequate. For others, additional help can come in the form of behavioral therapy and stress management. I do not believe this reflects any spiritual weakness or a lack of faith. To the contrary, through precept and example the Bible instructs us about the importance of seeking advice from wise people. This isn't "folk wisdom." There is scientific evidence showing that such counsel can protect the heart.

Restoring Peace

You will keep him in perfect peace, whose mind is stayed on You, because he trusts in You.
—ISAIAH 26:3

Whenever a person is under excessive psychosocial stress, especially if at high risk for cardiovascular disease, then some kind of stress management program can help. These are designed to reduce the impact of stress in several ways:

♥ Removing the source

♥ Changing our perception of it

♥ Reducing the adverse physiologic effects

♥ Learning to cope in ways that are not harmful

Stress management incorporates skills training with relaxation techniques. In some respects, handling stress effectively is a skill. If we learn how to do this, then the adverse effects will be diminished. Relaxation techniques can include such things as deep breathing, decreasing tension in the muscles, and retreating to a quiet environment. These measures can reduce the heart rate, lower the respiratory rate, and minimize muscle strain, which all reflect decreased sympathetic nervous system activity.

Physical activity and exercise are beneficial for stress reduction as well as optimizing control of anxiety disorders and depression. In one study, exercise coupled with stress management proved beneficial for those with cardiovascular disease. Investigators randomly assigned some 130 people with stable coronary artery disease to groups; among them were usual care, or usual care plus stress management. Compared to those receiving only usual care, those in the latter group had better heart function and enhanced blood flow to the heart in response to mental stress. They also scored better on surveys measuring general distress and depression.[20]

In addition to stress management and exercise, behavioral therapy is quite beneficial. For example, a group of Swedish investigators randomly assigned about 360 men and women recently discharged from the hospital following a heart attack or procedure (e.g., bypass surgery or angioplasty). Researchers placed them in one of two groups: (1) traditional care, or (2) traditional care plus cognitive behavioral therapy. The therapy sessions focused primarily on coping with stress. Held in twenty two-hour sessions over the course of a year, they were based on five key components: education, self-monitoring, skills training, cognitive restructuring, and spiritual development. Although participation in these sessions only lasted for a year, researchers followed the two groups for nearly eight years. Participants receiving traditional care and cognitive behavioral therapy (the Intervention group) had significantly fewer cardiac events, compared to those who received traditional care alone (the Reference group). And they realized benefits for years after completing the cognitive behavioral therapy sessions:[21]

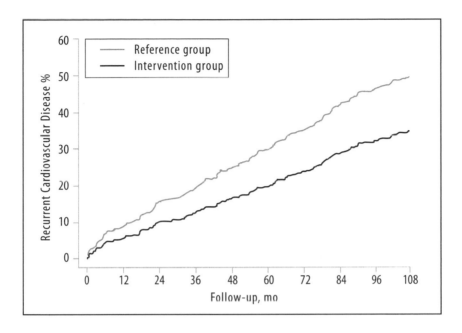

The Intervention group reported a 41 percent lower rate of fatal and nonfatal recurrent heart events, and 45 percent fewer heart attacks. This benefit increased in proportion to participation—men and women who attended the greatest number of sessions had the best outcomes.[22]

While this constitutes compelling evidence, it remains to be seen whether behavioral therapy and stress management courses will become standard treatment following a cardiac event. Will doctors and nurses one day prescribe behavioral therapy with the same frequency as aspirin or cholesterol-lowering medications? Only time will tell. As I mentioned, since research in this area is fairly new, it remains to be seen whether future standards of cardiac care will require a more systematic assessment of psychosocial variables. In the meantime, it should be clear that optimal heart health depends on how well we manifest the third fruit of the Holy Spirit: peace.

Chapter 6

DEPRESSION

I am troubled; I am bowed down greatly;
I go mourning all the day long.

Psalm 38:6, KJV

I F WE AREN'T CAREFUL, WE CAN FALL PREY TO THE SAME KIND of gloom that enveloped David when he felt as if God had forgotten him. Life's challenges can sometimes overwhelm us, including its seasons. From birth to death we move through phases—some short, others long. Life never stagnates, moving on in a continuing transformation. No matter how much we dislike change, it happens constantly. The seasons of nature parallel the aging process. Spring symbolizes birth. Summer represents growth. Autumn signifies middle age; just as leaves change color before falling from the trees, our hair changes color before falling off our head. Winter brings with it a bittersweet period of closure. We don't like to contemplate our mortality, but inevitably each of us will die.

In the decades-long transition from infancy to old age, the only constant is our identity. However, while who we are remains essentially the same, everything else is subject to change. Our values change. As we approach middle age, things we considered significant during childhood and adolescence become irrelevant. (This is one reason parenting is such a challenge. Connecting with our children requires that we recognize and validate matters that are important to them—even if we consider them trivial.) Our appearance changes too. The shape, size, and even the color of our bodies go through a steady state of transition. Muscles once firm go soft, taut skin relaxes, and formerly black or brown hair fades to silver or gray. Of course, there are ways to combat such changes, but that topic is beyond the scope of this book!

Certainly our moods vary from day to day. These fluctuations are more pronounced in women (no "amen" necessary, men!), in part because of cyclical shifts in our hormone levels. But neither gender always feels exactly the same. Some days we feel relaxed, and on others, irritable. Some days we are gregarious, while at other times we prefer solitude. On some days we feel happy, but on others sadness prevails. Solomon noted the inevitability of change when he wrote that there is "a time to weep, and a time to laugh; a time to mourn, and a time to dance" (Ecclesiastes 3:4). These subtle fluctuations in our moods represent a normal part of life—including sadness.

The Bible confirms this by showing us sadness (even profound sadness) in many leaders' lives, such as Jeremiah, the "weeping prophet." Jeremiah's people rejected God and refused to heed his warnings about the consequences of their rebellion: "But if you do not listen, I will weep in secret because of your pride; my eyes will weep bitterly, overflowing with tears, because the LORD's flock will be taken captive" (Jeremiah 13:17, NIV). After their brother, Lazarus, died, Mary and Martha experienced great sorrow. Knowing that Jesus could have intervened to prevent his death exacerbated their grief (John 11). Even Jesus came to the point of tears over the hardened hearts of the people of Israel: "As he approached Jerusalem and saw the city, he wept over it" (Luke 19:41, NIV).

Sadness is a part of life. Like any other mood or aspect of our being, it is subject to change. Life's experiences may bring sadness for a season, but then it dissipates. However, for some there is no obvious basis for sadness. Even worse, it fails to dissipate. When this occurs, sadness shifts from normalcy to pathology. What ought to be a temporary case of feeling low becomes a clinical state of depression.

Not Just "the Blues"

> For my days are consumed like smoke, and my bones are burned like a hearth. My heart is stricken and withered like grass, so that I forget to eat my bread. Because of the sound of my groaning my bones cling to my skin. I am like a pelican of the wilderness; I am like an owl of the desert. I lie awake, and am like a sparrow alone on the housetop.
>
> —Psalm 102:3–7

While temporary sadness is normal, clinical depression is not. Major depression falls under the category of "mood disorders." Unlike medical disorders that are typically diagnosed by specific test results (e.g., blood tests, biopsies, or X-rays), doctors diagnose psychiatric disorders based on whether or not a person has experienced or manifests specific criteria. Currently these criteria appear in the fourth edition of the *Diagnostic and Statistical Manual* (DSM-IV), released in 2000. (The fifth edition is due out in 2013.)

The writer of Psalm 102 may well have been depressed. Some Bible commentaries say the author felt great distress over the woes of Israel. Yet his words also sound a message of personal distress. Although we don't know how long he felt this way (a diagnosis of major depression incorporates duration as well as symptoms), his description meets several diagnostic criteria: (1) he is sad, (2) his sleep and appetite are disturbed, and (3) he gives the impression that he spends a great deal of time thinking about his mortality.

Doctors establish major depression when five or more of the following symptoms appear daily over a two-week period. They can be reported by the individual or observed by another person, such as a family member or a friend. At least one of the five symptoms must be from the first or second points (depressed mood or loss of interest).

♥ A depressed mood for most of the day, manifested as feeling sad, empty, apathetic, irritable, or indifferent

♥ A significantly reduced interest in activities or diminished pleasure when engaging in activities the person once considered enjoyable

♥ A decrease or increase in appetite, or a significant amount of weight loss (aside from the effects of dieting) or weight gain

♥ Insomnia or excessive sleep

♥ Feeling restless or feeling slowed down

♥ Loss of energy with fatigue nearly every day

♥ Feelings of excessive or inappropriate guilt or feelings of worthlessness

♥ Difficulty concentrating, inattentiveness, or indecisiveness

♥ Recurrent thoughts of death, thoughts of suicide (with or without a specific plan), or a suicide attempt

Other mood disorders include minor depression and dysthymic disorder, which is despondency or a tendency toward it. People with minor depression have fewer than the five symptoms required for a diagnosis of major depression. Or if they experience five or more, their frequency is not as constant. (Symptoms may be intermittent rather than on consecutive days or occur for only a short time each day.)

People with dysthymic disorder exhibit symptoms that are not quite as incapacitating as those found with major depression. Yet they are present for a long time—at least two years. With dysthymic disorder feelings of sadness are present most days for the majority of the day and are accompanied by at least two of the following:

- ♥ Change in appetite (decreased or increased)

- ♥ Change in sleep (insomnia or excessive sleep)

- ♥ Poor concentration

- ♥ Low self-esteem

- ♥ Low energy

- ♥ Hopelessness

To be sure, there is overlap between various mood disorders; in terms of a specific diagnosis, many "gray zones" exist. I want to specifically mention bipolar disorder, mainly because many people who are diagnosed as depressed—even treated for it—have bipolar disorder. With this condition depressed moods are interspersed with periods of mood elevation. It is important to make this distinction, especially since the treatment differs. However, here I will focus primarily on major depression.

Despite modern medical advances, doctors have not clearly defined an underlying cause for major depression. Several variables, both internal and external, are likely to play a role in its onset. Studies on the incidence of depression in twins and families confirm a genetic link. Experiencing adversity early in life (such as child abuse or child neglect) will increase the likelihood for future bouts with depression. There is also strong evidence confirming a disturbance or imbalance in several brain chemicals—specifically serotonin, norepinephrine, and dopamine. Some of the most effective medications used to treat depression work by modifying the effects of these chemicals.

Approximately 17 percent of the population will experience an episode of major depression at some point in their lives. Depression is a leading cause of disability worldwide and is currently one of the ten most important global health statistics, according to the World Health Organization. This agency estimates that by the year 2020 it will rank second only to cardiac disease with respect to degree of disability.[1]

Compared with men, depression is nearly twice as common in women, and more common in whites compared to blacks. However, among blacks it tends to be more chronic and is associated with a greater degree of functional impairment. While the prevalence of depression declines with age, certain groups of elderly individuals—those with chronic medical illnesses and residents of assisted living or skilled nursing facilities—have a greater degree of depression, compared to younger adults. Although life's trials can precipitate depression, its onset is not necessarily contingent upon life's circumstances. In other words, life doesn't have to *be* bad in order for a person to *feel* bad.

With regard to establishing a diagnosis in a timely manner, depression is similar to type 2 diabetes. As with diabetes, many people who are depressed will dismiss their symptoms or attribute them to another cause. To make matters worse, physicians who are not psychiatrists may miss the diagnosis in more than half of the patients who come into their offices in a depressed state.[2] This is partially due to the fact that depression can cause such physical symptoms as fatigue and body aches. Thus the problem can go unrecognized (by patient and health care provider) and untreated for long periods of time—even years.

Depression is a disorder that gives evidence of the connection between mind and body. People with depression are more likely to develop disease in their physical body (including heart disease). Those with chronic medical illnesses, including heart disease, are more susceptible to depression. In fact, the prevalence of major depression is estimated to be as high as 20 percent in people with such chronic conditions as diabetes and heart disease. When depression and chronic medical illnesses coexist, it adversely affects outcomes of controlling the disease, mortality rate, and health care costs.

Its costs are enormous. Medical expenses of depression associated with chronic medical illness are approximately 50 percent higher, regardless of the severity of the chronic illness.[3] In the United States, the cost of depression (incorporating higher health care utilization and diminished productivity in the workplace) is estimated at $83 billion annually.[4] A 2007 study that assessed the health of nearly two hundred fifty thousand participants from sixty countries showed that depression had a significantly greater effect on declining health (and thus medical expenses), compared with arthritis, asthma, diabetes, or angina.[5]

So why does depression exacerbate physical illness? Several factors play a role, notably that its effects are not limited to the realm of the mind. Depression leads to measurable physiologic changes within the body. In addition, there are many components to chronic illness, which people experience in varying degrees. Pain, disability, the need for continuous self-care, having to depend on others, and even a sense of losing control are just some of the "extras" accompanying chronic medical conditions. People with depression are less equipped to cope with such major life adjustments.

Likewise, changing the diet, increasing physical activity, following a strict schedule for multiple medications, and showing up consistently for office visits requires considerable motivation, enthusiasm, focus, and commitment. While necessary for optimal care, all are depleted by depression. Finally, depressed people are at a higher risk for engaging in such detrimental habits as smoking, excessive drinking, and illicit drug use. To add insult to injury, even those who want to break these bad habits find it especially difficult to do so. This connection between depression and all forms of physical illness includes an impact on the cardiovascular system.

Depression and Cardiovascular Disease

The troubles of my heart have enlarged; bring me out of my distresses!

—PSALM 25:17

For several decades clinical researchers have more closely examined the link between heart disease and depression. The connection has been recognized for centuries—even during biblical times. Scientific evidence gathered more recently augments what we have long known through intuition and random observation. And it reveals a two-edged sword. Not only are those with depression more susceptible to heart disease, but also people with heart disease are more likely to get depressed. Depression is about three times more common in patients after a heart attack than in the general community.[6]

In addition, assessments on patients hospitalized for heart attacks show that 15 to 20 percent meet the diagnostic criteria for major depression.[7] If that weren't bad enough, depression is associated with an earlier onset of heart disease and a worsened prognosis. As the severity of depression increases, so does the severity of heart disease, irrespective of other risk factors like diabetes and hypertension.

What might explain this connection—biologically? While the cause remains unclear, people with depression (compared with those who are not depressed) are more likely to have physiologic changes associated with heart disease. Various abnormalities have been detected in people with depression. They include such factors as a decline in the variability of heart rate, higher levels of inflammatory markers (e.g., C-reactive protein, interleukin-6, and fibrinogen), increased platelet aggregation, impaired endothelial function, and unfavorable changes in glucose regulation. All can potentially contribute to the onset or aggravation of heart disease.

Lifestyle also plays a powerful role; behavioral changes resulting from a depressed mood are a key determinant in this association. For example, the Heart and Soul Study assessed more than one thousand participants with stable coronary artery disease for depression. The findings showed a significant association between depressive symptoms and heart disease. Participants who were depressed had a 50 percent higher rate of heart attack, stroke, heart failure, or death than those who were not depressed. When investigators teased out the contribution of behaviors associated with depression—particularly low levels of exercise and physical activity—the association between depression and heart disease greatly diminished.[8]

The Cardiovascular Health Study further confirmed this. It followed close to six thousand elderly people for approximately a decade. Not surprisingly, participants with high depression scores faced an increased risk for death from heart disease. However, investigators learned that a low level of physical activity accounted for about 25 percent of this increased risk.[9]

Depression also aggravates sleep conditions. People with depression are more prone to insomnia; poor sleep habits have been linked to heart disease. While the connection is not clear, experimental studies show that sleep deprivation leads to increases in the levels of inflammatory markers in the blood. These same markers are associated with cardiovascular disease.[10] However, it remains to be determined whether sleep deprivation contributes to excessive heart disease risk—and if so, to what extent.

So questions remain with regard to the heart disease-mood disorder connection. Does it rest primarily in physiologic disturbances (such as changes in the heart rate, endothelial cells, and chemicals in the bloodstream)? Or does it stem from a diminished capacity from someone suffering with depression to follow a "heart-healthy" lifestyle, including adequate exercise, a proper diet, sufficient sleep, regular checkups, and adherence to medications? More than likely both contribute to different degrees in different individuals. Whatever the case may be, the bottom line is that the connection is real—depression poses a serious risk for the development of cardio-vascular disease, as well as its outcomes.

The Women's Health Initiative examined this connection, screening nearly ninety-four thousand women ages fifty to seventy-nine for depression and following them for four years. Approximately 16 percent had initial scores that indicated depression; 12 percent had at least one bout with past depression. Researchers found that depression (past or present) increased the risk of death from heart disease among women who did not have any apparent heart disease at the start of the study. In these women depression represented an independent risk factor. Its effect was separate from others, such as age, smoking, body weight, physical activity, high cholesterol, diabetes, and hypertension.[11]

Not only is there a connection between heart disease and depression, but also people with depression have poorer outcomes following a cardiac event (including surgery) compared with those not suffering from depression. In one study, researchers assessed depression among more than three hundred patients soon after coronary artery bypass surgery. Approximately 20 percent met the criteria for major depression. Over the next ten years sixty-two of the original group died from heart disease. Three factors proved independent risks for death: age, strength of the heart (how well the heart contracted), and whether they met the criteria for major depression.[12]

With this connection between heart disease and depression, it becomes prudent—even life-preserving—to screen for and acknowledge the signs of depression. What patients and their doctors should not do is ignore or make light of the symptoms. Doing so puts the mind in jeopardy as well as the body, particularly the heart. Don't be afraid to take the proverbial "bull by the horns" and confront common mood disorders. There are many approaches to therapy to treat these problems.

Approach to Treatment

…but your sorrow will be turned into joy.

—John 16:20

At the Last Supper Jesus told His disciples He would be going away, but He promised that the Holy Spirit ("the Helper") would come after His departure. Being fully human and thereby connecting with human nature, Jesus knew they would respond with sadness: "But because I have said these things to you, sorrow has filled your heart" (John 16:6). Not only would the disciples experience intense grief after His death, but they would also face severe persecution after His crucifixion. In some cases this would include martyrdom: "They will put you out of the synagogues; yes, the time is coming that whoever kills you will think that he offers God service" (verse 2).

Grief and stressful conditions provide the perfect milieu for depression. This is exactly what lay in store for the disciples. It is quite interesting that Jesus, who loved them with an unfathomable love, didn't mention the option of changing their circumstances to more placid conditions. While never promising good times, He assured them their sorrow would turn to joy. This reminds us that the joy of the Lord is not contingent on life's circumstances, and it attests to the truth that God's loves for us is infallible—even in the midst of adversity. Despite grief and adversity in our lives, we too can be filled with joy.

As a follower of Christ I believe the first approach to treating depression is to grow in this fruit of the Holy Spirit. Joy sustains us, comforts us, and gives us hope. However, as a physician, I also understand we live in a fallen world. This means from birth we face death, disability, and all manner of diseases. Some affect the body, and others, the mind. Unfortunately a stigma attaches to mental illness that generally doesn't exist with physical disease. Misconceptions persist that mental illness is shameful, best ignored, or that we should just "get over it." Such stigmata are especially prevalent in the church. As a result, many local congregations become places of silent suffering. Depression prevails, but people avoid effective therapy because they fear rejection or—worse yet—being considered unbiblical. I have observed encouraging signs lately; many congregations are devoting attention to mental health, particularly depression. Although much work remains, we are making progress toward eliminating the shame associated with psychiatric disorders.

There are methods for treating and controlling depression, particularly medications and psychotherapy. In the rest of this chapter I will also examine how relationships impact our mental health, as well as take a closer look at the power of joy.

Medications and Psychotherapy

Therefore remove sorrow from your heart...
                                    —ECCLESIASTES 11:10

In cases of major depression, the initial choice of treatment depends on the severity of the symptoms. Those with mild to moderate depression benefit equally from either psychotherapy or medications, although medications bring about remission more quickly. In cases of mild to moderate disease, combining psychotherapy and medications has not proven superior. However, in cases of severe depression, combining the two has yielded the best results.

The vast majority of people with depression can be treated in an outpatient setting. However, some cases (for example, suicidal thoughts) warrant hospitalization. Effective psychotherapy treatments for depression include cognitive, interpersonal, and problem solving. As noted, with mild to moderate illness all three are as effective as medications; some studies show psychotherapy offers more protection against relapse. Personal preference should factor into the choice between the two, with the stipulation it be based on a clear, accurate understanding of each. In one study people who mistakenly believed that medications used for treating depression led to addiction were more likely to choose psychotherapy.[13]

All forms of psychotherapy require a great degree of training. Consequently, such treatment may not be as readily accessible—especially in rural areas—as medications. In addition, insurance plans may place restrictions on types that qualify for reimbursement. Remember that psychotherapy must be administered by *trained professionals*. While simply talking to a friend, a family member, or even a pastor might make you feel better, it does not necessarily constitute psychotherapy.

Most medications used to treat depression modify the action of various chemicals in the brain. For others, including St. John's wort (an herbal treatment for depression), the way they work is not entirely clear. While a detailed description of approved medications would take too much space, generally they fall into the following categories:

- ♥ Selective serotonin reuptake inhibitors (SSRIs)

- ♥ Serotonin and norepinephrine reuptake inhibitors (SNRIs)

- ♥ Tricyclic antidepressants (TCAs)

- ♥ Monoamine oxidase inhibitors (MAOs)

- ♥ Others, including dopamine reuptake inhibitors, 5-HT$_2$ receptor antagonists, norepinephrine uptake inhibitors, and St. John's wort

When a medication is deemed appropriate, its selection revolves around such factors as side effects, interactions with other medications, whether the patient has taken it before, and its effectiveness, along with cost and insurance coverage. The goal of therapy is complete remission and a return to normal functioning. If the first medication selected doesn't work, options include switching to a different drug, adding a second prescription, adding psychotherapy, or switching to psychotherapy. Once a patient achieves remission, he or she should continue the medication for an additional four to nine months—or longer for the elderly and those with chronic medical illnesses.

Recognize that medications used to treat depression don't work instantly. When I prescribe them, I warn patients that antidepressants will not work like pain medications that typically provide noticeable relief within an hour or so. To the contrary, the drug may take a week—sometimes as long as a month—before the patient feels any different. People should take antidepressants each day and continue them even after depressive symptoms fade. Never discontinue them without checking first with your doctor or other health care provider.

Patients who see depression resurface after stopping a medication should resume and maintain it for a longer period of time. In some cases, such as multiple recurrences or severe depression, lifelong therapy may be the best approach. Psychotherapy may be a better choice for adolescents and pregnant women, where the risks of medications can outweigh the benefits. As with all chronic illnesses, social support plays a vital role.

Relationships and Support Systems

> Then the women said to Naomi, "Blessed be the LORD, who has not left you this day without a close relative."
> —RUTH 4:14

There is a strong connection between health and relationships—in both a positive and negative sense. Good relationships promote good health and a positive mental outlook; bad relationships can harm them. Once again, scientific studies have confirmed what we have known intuitively and through years of informal observation: the strength and quality of our social networks have a direct influence on the risk of disease, including depression and cardiovascular disease.

In this technologically advanced era I need to clarify what I mean by a "social network." I am not referring to electronic connections like Facebook or Twitter, where one might have thousands of "friends" and "followers" yet still feel isolated and lonely. I use the term in a traditional sense—meaning quality, face-to-face, flesh-and-blood relationships with family, friends, and community. Texting dozens of buddies about the latest music group or political controversy doesn't qualify.

Before looking at scientific evidence, I will examine a biblical case in point—the account of Ruth and Naomi. If you are not familiar with the story of these two women, I encourage you to pause, grab a Bible, and read the Book of Ruth. Just four chapters long, this sweet story contains a rich review of biblical history and precepts of the Christian faith.

Naomi, her husband, and their two sons traveled to Moab to escape a famine in her homeland of Bethlehem in Judah. While there, her sons married Moabite women named Ruth and Orpah. In this foreign country Naomi's social network consisted of her husband, her two sons, and their wives. Then calamity struck; all three men died. Afterward Naomi decided to return to her native land with her two daughters-in-law. However, ultimately only Ruth stayed with her.

This meant Naomi's social network unexpectedly dwindled from five individuals to one. To make matters worse, she lost the key men in her life in a culture and era where a woman needed a male "covering" (e.g., a father, husband, or son) for provision and protection. Such a system left widows and single women at an extreme disadvantage. Being in a foreign land isolated Naomi in many respects:

♥ The distance separating her from her homeland

♥ Ethnic differences between her background and the Moabite language, customs, and food

♥ Moab represented a place of spiritual isolation. Moabites did not worship the God of Israel.

♥ To compound her problems, Naomi had no convenient means of connecting with friends and family back in Judah. The multiple ways to communicate that we often take for granted (letters, phone calls, e-mail, Skype, and texting) were not an option.

This change in circumstances ushered in grief, uncertainty, and isolation, which had a profound effect on her sense of well-being. At the close of chapter one, when she and Ruth arrive in Judah, Naomi gives a revealing self-assessment:

> Now the two of them went until they came to Bethlehem. And it happened, when they had come to Bethlehem, that all the city was excited because of them; and the women said, "Is this Naomi?" But she said to them, "Do not call me Naomi; call me Mara, for the Almighty has dealt very bitterly with me. I went out full, and the LORD has brought me home again empty. Why do you call me Naomi, since the LORD has testified against me, and the Almighty has afflicted me?"
> —RUTH 1:19–21

Although *Naomi* means "pleasant," we can see her rejecting the name because of the *un*pleasantness of her condition. She asks to be called "Mara," meaning "bitter." In her estimation this name better describes who she had become. The close of chapter 1 certainly marks a low point in Naomi's life. However, by the end of the book her joy returns. This path to restoration begins in chapter 2, when she reconnects with her social network—family, friends, and community in Bethlehem.

While chapter 1 concludes with words reflecting a bitter heart, chapter 2 begins: "There was a *relative* of Naomi's husband..." (Ruth 2:1, emphasis added). Thus starts the healing process, a transition that attests to the power of social networks and the role that relatives play in our mental and physical well-being. Both the quantity and quality of our relationships impact our health. The reason I included the previous disclaimers about electronic "friends" is that while *quantity* may number in the thousands, *quality* is often missing. In addition, our relationships can be categorized (e.g., children, neighbors, classmates), with each offering a distinct resource.

For instance, an elderly person may have a spouse or close friend who provides emotional support, siblings offering financial support, and children contributing such services as transportation and housekeeping. The quality of our relationships affects the status of our physical health more than the number of people we know. In fact, a satisfactory support system can even change our perception of well-being. Responses from the elderly in the National Health and Nutrition Examination Survey demonstrated this. Regardless of race or gender, older people who considered their support system inadequate were twice as likely to classify themselves as having poor health, compared to those who were satisfied with their social networks.[14]

The biblical account of Naomi provides a vivid picture of her emotional health. However, other than being able to complete the journey back to Judah, we don't know much about her physical condition. With respect to the impact on mental and emotional well-being, hundreds of scientific studies examining social networks have yielded results that line up with Naomi's pleasant experience. However, studies have also shown a strong connection between social networks and physical health, including the risk for cardiovascular disease.

Some risk factors and behaviors that will increase the chance for heart disease are often clustered in social groups. For example, people who smoke tend to associate with other smokers. Likewise, people in our social circle influence our body weight. One study found that an individual's chance of becoming obese increased by 57 percent if a good friend became obese, compared to only 40 percent if a sibling became obese and 37 percent if one's spouse became obese.[15]

While our social network has the capacity to influence habits and lifestyles, close relationships also exert an independent, stronger impact on health. In a large study conducted by the Harvard School of Public Health, more than thirty-two thousand male health professionals who were free of cardiovascular disease were assessed for—among other things—the strength of their social ties. Researchers found that over the course of four years the socially isolated (single, fewer than six friends or relatives, and no church or community group affiliations) were more likely to die from cardiovascular disease than men with stronger social networks.[16]

Relationships, depression, and heart disease are so intertwined that each influences the other to some degree. Depression impacts relationships, and relationships can either protect against or contribute to the development of depression. In turn, both have a direct influence on chronic conditions like cardiovascular disease. Heart disease management requires lifestyle modification, whose long-term success is hindered by depression and a lack of social support—and so forth.

For depressed women, researchers found that just the thought of a person within their social network had an impact on their heart. They monitored blood pressure response in depressed and nondepressed women after asking both groups to think about a person with whom they had a close relationship. They found depressed women experienced a rise in blood pressure. Among women who were not depressed, blood pressure decreased.[17] Without question, the quality of our social ties plays a major role in depression and cardiovascular disease. Our relationships provide emotional support, financial support, encouragement, and assistance with decision-making and daily tasks. Best of all, our relationships have the capacity to magnify our joy.

Smile, Laugh, Shout for Joy!

Make a joyful noise unto the LORD, all ye lands. Serve the LORD with gladness: come before his presence with singing.
—PSALM 100:1–2, KJV

Joy is the second fruit of the Holy Spirit listed in Galatians 5:22. None of the Spirit's attributes are conditional. That means that the joy of the Lord is ours. Regardless of life's circumstances, and whether sad or gloomy, joy can still reign. The same is true amid troubles and hardships, even financial strains that accompanied the extended economic downturn that began in 2007. It is a blessing to experience the joy of the Holy Spirit when we feel somber. But—praise the Lord—it is a blessing indeed when His joy ushers feelings of gladness into our hearts.

In chapter 4 I looked at how our disposition (positive or negative) can affect our health. Thus far in this chapter I have examined the connection between depression and cardiovascular disease and reviewed the important role that relationships and social networks play in our overall well-being. I will conclude with a look at what I call a *corporate* disposition, meaning the way we feel is significantly influenced by the mood of those close to us. While we ought to strive to maintain a positive disposition, it is vital to guard against being swayed by naysayers around us.

Happiness spreads from person to person. Framingham Heart Study researchers learned this by following nearly five thousand participants for more than twenty years. They discovered that happiness, like obesity and the tendency to smoke, was a collective phenomenon. In this particular segment of the study a person's happiness extended up to three degrees of separation. In other words, an individual's happiness was affected by whether (or not) the friends of one's friends' friends were happy! Their findings revealed that "pockets" of happiness did not develop because happy people tend to associate with others like them. They stemmed from happiness *spreading* from person to person. If someone had a friend living within a mile, and that friend became happy, the first person's happiness increased by 25 percent. This was the case for siblings who lived within a mile of each other, spouses, and next-door neighbors. This effect did not appear among coworkers and diminished with time and longer geographical distances.[18]

This is just one example of the benefits of associating with happy people. Given these scientific findings, I find it interesting that nearly two thousand years ago the writer of the book of Hebrews gave this directive: "Let us not give up meeting together, as some are in the habit of doing, but let us encourage one another—and all the more as you see the Day approaching" (Hebrews 10:25, NIV). In other words, we should attend church regularly and not skip services. Watching a Christian TV program does not constitute "meeting together" and cannot provide the benefits of corporate worship. In addition to mutual encouragement, we benefit from collective prayer, fellowship, and growing together in wisdom and knowledge. Another great reward in coming together is demonstrated by the Framingham Heart Study: spreading happiness.

The psalmist speaks to this in Psalm 100. When God's people assembled together, a cheerful spirit flowed through the congregation. In Old Testament times God's presence brought joy, which was manifested in a spirit of gladness. Even entering the place of worship uplifted the soul: "Enter into His gates with thanksgiving, and into His courts with praise" (Psalm 100:4). This atmosphere of gladness appeared in the first-century church as well, although by then God lived in the hearts of believers through His indwelling Spirit: "So continuing daily with one accord in the temple, and breaking bread from house to house, they ate their food with gladness and simplicity of heart" (Acts 2:46).

Once again this shows the connection between body, mind, and spirit. Being in the presence of God's people spreads gladness. Not only does this joy protect against depression, but also it has the potential to lower our risk for cardiovascular disease. This shows the wisdom inherent in Hebrews' admonition to not forsake assembling together. It also reminds us of other directives in Scripture to keep God's commandments, such as the verse reminding us that "His commandments are not burdensome" (1 John 5:3). The command to assemble together is not a burden, bringing with it the blessing of better health.

It is a tragedy that some people avoid church or have forsaken it because their congregations weren't governed by God's Spirit but by fleshly, self-centered spirits. In many churches joy and gladness are not evident. If that describes yours, don't throw the baby out with the bathwater! Don't give up because of a problem; become part of the solution. Let your light shine, commit yourself to prayer, and love unconditionally; there is much power in all of these. And never stop believing that God is able to transform what we think is *our* church into *His* church, the kind of place where joy flows freely and blesses abundantly—physically, mentally, and spiritually.

Chapter 7

CURBING ANGER

Let all bitterness, wrath, anger, clamor, and evil
speaking be put away from you, with all malice.
And be kind to one another, tenderhearted, forgiving
one another, just as God in Christ forgave you.

Ephesians 4:31–32

IT'S THE KIND OF AMUSING EXPLOSION MADE POPULAR BY "MAD
scientist" movies. After the wild-eyed protagonist mixes a strange
elixir that contains some kind of acid, gas and smoke pour from a
Pyrex bottle, followed by bubbles forming on a countertop and part
of the surface vanishing before a huge *bang!* erupts. Yet encounters
with acid are no laughing matter. Anyone who took Chemistry 101
in college—or a basic course in high school—learned something
about acids. A strong acid with a low pH can destroy on contact.
If that happens to be your skin, intense pain follows. Unless the
acid is quickly neutralized, its caustic effects continue after initial
contact.

Just as acid can permanently transform whatever it touches,
the acidic emotion of anger can destroy and alter everything in its
path. Uncontrolled, misdirected, and selfishly motivated anger not
only harms the object of its wrath, but it also damages the source.
Anger injures the angry person's physical, mental, and emotional

health—that is, the self-centered variety. So, not all anger is bad, just the misdirected kind.

The same is true of acid. For instance, stomach acid is essential to digestion. Without it, our bodies can't break down the foods we eat and transfer their nutrients into our bloodstream. However, if the stomach produces an excessive amount of acid, or if acid goes beyond its boundaries and travels into the esophagus, problems follow. Anyone who has suffered with heartburn from acid reflux can attest to such pain.

So, acid is beneficial when confined to its proper place and restricted to appropriate conditions. Likewise, properly manifested anger is good. God has the capacity for wrath. (See Psalm 89:46; Romans 1:18; Revelation 6:15-17.) Jesus demonstrated a great measure of anger when He cleansed the temple (John 2:13–17). Such righteous indignation shows that the difference between "good" and "bad" anger rests with the heart's motivation and intent.

Unlike ungodly anger, righteous anger is never uncontrolled, misdirected, or selfish. While God's wrath churns up in response to sin, He always controls it. Remember that His nature includes self-control, the ninth fruit of the Holy Spirit listed in Galatians 5:22–23. Ungodly anger typically manifests itself in response to a personal insult, whether real or imagined. It is self-centered and out of control (a reliable indicator of ungodliness). This is the anger Paul addressed in the passage from Ephesians 4 that opened this chapter.

As with other emotions, the person who feels ungodly anger tends to think it is beyond his or her ability to control. We even spout clichés to convince ourselves that unharnessed, anger-driven speech justifies our behavior:

- ♥ "What comes up, comes out."

- ♥ "I just call them as I see them."

- ♥ "Well, I needed to get that off my chest."

We can even persuade ourselves that we are not being true to ourselves or may even harm ourselves if we don't release internal rage in all its fury. However, such notions are contrary to Scripture. When Paul told us to put away such toxic emotions as anger, wrath, malice, and bitterness, he meant just that. *Get rid of them!* We ought not to spread them to everyone around us, whether the source of the offense or an innocent bystander. Nor should we take anger deep in our soul and nurture the kind of bitter roots that will mature into bitter fruit, or refresh and rehearse offenses repeatedly in our minds, for weeks or months at a time. Instead we are to put them away. That means we process them, subject them to God's Word, and eliminate them in obedience to God. Now, I'm not saying this is easy. Through thoughtless or careless words or insensitive actions other people can inflict deep wounds. However, we must learn to discipline our reactions. When we resist Paul's directions to put anger away, we place ourselves at risk for destruction.

Angry thoughts and feelings are fair game for anyone. No matter what your underlying nature, at some time or another everyone has likely gotten provoked to the point of demonstrating uncontrolled, selfish anger. Whether it was simply a sarcastic remark mumbled under our breath or a fit of violent rage, we can remember an instance when anger got the best of us. Although anger can rear its ugly head in anybody's life, some people are more susceptible. They may have a relatively stable personality when all is going smooth. However, if they get offended, they react with more intensity and a higher degree of rage. In addition, their anger tends to remain "fresh" longer.

This means anger typically falls into two categories: (1) intermittent episodes that most of us are liable to exhibit from time to time, and (2) "trait anger," which is the volatile personality I just described. A warning: both are linked to cardiovascular disease. I will start with an exploration of trait anger.

The Angry Disposition

And Cain was very angry, and his countenance fell.

—Genesis 4:5

Before examining the heart connection, I need to elaborate a bit more on anger, which is manifested in two forms—active and passive.

Active anger erupts in such outward forms as yelling, loud arguing, using words with the intent to hurt, fighting, and damaging property. The worst form ultimately manifests itself in murder. Modern-day highway incidents turned deadly gave rise to the term "road rage." After a number of shooting incidents involving current or former postal employees, some coined the phrase "going postal" to describe outbursts of anger in the workplace. And while Cain exhibited active anger in killing his brother Abel, he also demonstrated a tendency toward passive anger.

The latter appears in Genesis 4:5; though he was very angry, the only manifestation surfaced through Cain's facial expression. Some might argue that a scowl (a "fallen countenance") is active anger, not passive. That is a good point, since facial expressions and body language are effective forms of communication. Even without sharp words, maintaining a specific demeanor to convey an angry message is an active choice. The countenance speaks volumes; although not destroying a person's property or life, it can inflict wounds more harmful than physical blows.

This is where learning to discipline ourselves and taming angry outbursts can pay long-term dividends, both with personal relationships and physical health. As Solomon said, "Wisdom brightens a man's face and changes its hard appearance" (Ecclesiastes 8:1, NIV). In the biblical sense, fools are predisposed to anger. But when they embrace wisdom, foolishness and ungodly anger will cease. Their facial expression follows suit, going from "hard" to "bright."

Cain exhibited a hard face, even before he murdered his brother. People with passive anger might not say or do anything and still harbor destructive anger. Unlike Cain, whose face gave a reliable clue to his inner feelings, someone with passive anger often wears a neutral demeanor. Their outward disposition may even appear pleasant as they behave with a surface, sugary kindness that takes hypocrisy to the extreme.

Passive anger, particularly in marriage, commonly manifests itself in "the silent treatment." One spouse offers either no response or a curt reply, or a bland, disinterested comment. Whether the passive person is your spouse, friend, or coworker, under normal circumstances this person may be an engaging conversationalist. When provoked, though, their passive anger surfaces in single-word answers or curt replies. It usually isn't helpful to point out this shortcoming, since they will justify their selfish actions to the bitter end: "Nothing is wrong; I answered your question, didn't I?"

Passive anger also surfaces through actions—or more often, a lack of action. Take the once-cooperative team player at work who is suddenly not available or doesn't participate with any measure of enthusiasm. This individual's withdrawal might sabotage an important project, just when the rest of the staff is working feverishly against a tight deadline. At home the passively angry person can disrupt household operations—no clean underwear to wear in the morning or dinner prepared in the evening. These angry folks shrug that they couldn't find time to wash clothes or shop for groceries. Again, confronting this passive anger is usually an exercise in futility: "What do you mean! I AM helping out on this project!" or, "Give me a break; I'm not perfect! Can't I forget to do the laundry?"

Damaging the Heart

Whether active or passive, and whether episodic or chronic, anger negatively impacts the heart. People with chronic anger as a personality trait are at a particularly high risk. Certainly their hearts are subject to the immediate consequences of intermittent outbursts of anger. However, many scientific studies have confirmed the heightened risks for cardiovascular disease in people with anger as a trait of their personality. This is in addition to the risk they incur from periodic outbursts.

A study done in 2000 examined the connection between anger trait and the outcomes of heart attack, death from heart disease, or the need for an invasive procedure to restore the heart's circulation. Of nearly thirteen thousand participants (both male and female, and African American and white), those with a normal blood pressure but a personality characterized by anger had a greater risk for all measurable heart disease outcomes than those with a normal blood pressure and low anger trait.[1]

In the Veterans Administration Normative Aging Study, a group of approximately thirteen hundred older veterans with no evidence of coronary heart disease completed a personality inventory that assessed (among other variables) the way they handled anger. Researchers categorized participants based on problems controlling anger and then followed them for an average span of seven years. During this interval several veterans manifested some form of heart disease, including heart attacks and angina; some died from heart disease. While not surprising given their age and the prevalence of cardiovascular disease in men, an interesting association between heart disease and anger surfaced. Men who reported the highest level of anger trait had a risk for a coronary event three times greater than men reporting the lowest levels.[2]

In a similar study, researchers assessed nearly two thousand middle-aged men without coronary heart disease using a personality inventory to score their level of hostility. Over the next ten years men with lower hostility scores showed a smaller risk for a major heart event than men with high scores. Interestingly, twenty years after the initial assessment, investigators found that men with high hostility scores were at an increased risk for not only heart disease but also death from any cause, including cancer.[3]

While these three studies looked primarily at older adults, evidence of the deleterious effects of trait anger can appear at a relatively young age. One study followed nearly eleven hundred young, male medical students for an average of thirty-six years. Participants completed a questionnaire that ascertained their reactions to stressful conditions. Over the next three-plus decades, these students-turned-physicians who exhibited the highest levels of anger during medical school showed a significantly greater risk for developing heart disease (particularly heart attacks) before the age of fifty-five.[4]

In his letter to the church in Ephesus, Paul quoted the Old Testament, reminding the Ephesians (and by extension, us) to "be angry, and do not sin"; he followed with the advice, "Do not let the sun go down on your wrath, nor give place to the devil" (Ephesians 4:26–27). Those with an angry personality trait let the sun repeatedly go down on their wrath. Their round-the-clock nature reveals some feature of anger, whether expressed as cynicism, bitterness, hostility, discontentment, complaining, pessimism, irritation, or paranoia.

The studies I just referenced should not surprise us, since they confirm the truth of God's Word. John 10:10 says, "The thief does not come except to steal, and to kill, and to destroy." The thief is the devil. When we allow anger to define us, harbor it in our souls, and integrate it into our persona, we must understand this choice includes clearly defined consequences. "Giving place" to the devil means facilitating his presence by following fleshly human impulses and venting our anger. This makes it easier for his plans to succeed, including his objectives of destroying and killing. (For those who think such language is extreme, explain the destruction of millions of American households by anger-induced divorces.) For those persons with an angry personality trait, the devil achieves this fatal objective quite commonly via the heart.

Sporadic Anger

> Now Naaman, commander of the army of the king of Syria, was a great and honorable man in the eyes of his master, because by him the LORD had given victory to Syria. He was also a mighty man of valor, but a leper.
>
> —2 KINGS 5:1

Chronic anger poses a risk to the heart, but there is also a risk in sporadic outbursts of anger, even for those without an angry personality. While the scientific evidence validating the link is fairly recent, mankind has observed this connection or suspected it intuitively for centuries.

As I mentioned in an earlier chapter, the Bible teaches by precept and example. It lists specific things we should do and things to avoid, or it provides an account of someone's life to use as a learning tool. The story of Naaman—commander of the Syrian army—and the Israeli prophet Elisha offers a good example of the latter. This story teaches that an impulsive outburst of anger has the potential to destroy.

Scripture introduces Naaman in 2 Kings 5. The start of the chapter records some of his positive attributes: a high military rank, his master's admiration, and his description as a "mighty man of valor," which speaks to his courage, loyalty, and expertise. However, he also had leprosy, a serious skin disease. Typically shunned by most of society, lepers had strong motivation to find help. So when Naaman learned from a young Israelite girl that a prophet living in Samaria could heal him, he arranged a visit.

This great warrior arrived at the prophet's house with an

entourage of horses and chariots. Although Elisha knew a high-ranking official was at his door, instead of stepping outside for a formal introduction, he dispatched a messenger to give Naaman specific (albeit brief) instructions on what to do for his leprosy. Not expecting such a curt and rather undignified reception, "Naaman became furious" (verse 11). Angry that Elisha did not come outside, he also took issue with his message to wash in the Jordan River. After all, Naaman thought, the Abanah and Pharpar rivers in Damascus were much better than anything in Israel. (He reminds me of some patients who are convinced that brand-name medications are superior to generics, a fallacy influenced heavily by TV advertising.)

Naaman came close to allowing anger to sabotage an opportunity for healing. At the height of his offense, "he turned and went away in a rage" (verse 12). This offers a clue as to why the Bible says chronically angry people are fools. Imagine Naaman, prepared to leave the very place he came to find healing, just as leprous as when he arrived! All because he allowed sporadic anger to get the best of him. Fortunately, anger didn't prevent him from listening to reason. When his servant spoke rationally and told Naaman he would have followed more complex instructions, Naaman calmed down. And, after bathing in the Jordan River, the Syrian commander was healed. This is evidence that Naaman did not have an angry personality trait. People with such chronic anger do not see the error of their ways, nor do they respond with any humility. A chronically angry person would have rounded up all his chariots, feeling fully justified in rejecting Elisha's advice, and returned to Syria to spend the rest of his days blaming the prophet for his leprous skin.

However, while chronic anger carries serious health consequences, sporadic anger also proves detrimental to the heart. There are physiologic reasons for this. Heart attacks, angina, and sudden cardiac death follow a circadian pattern, meaning they take place in rhythmic biological cycles that recur at approximately twenty-four-hour intervals. The peak incidence of heart-related problems occurs between 6:00 a.m. and noon.[5]

In the morning our sympathetic nervous system releases various chemicals to stir things up to help us wake up and start the day. This increases our blood pressure and heart rate. Our heart begins to consume more oxygen than required during deep sleep. For most people, the heart handles these morning shifts uneventfully. However, for others—particularly those at risk for heart disease— this early-morning stress may be significant enough to cause problems. The relationship? Anger also stimulates the sympathetic nervous system, causing a surge of the same hormones released during the early morning hours. So the same mechanism responsible for a disproportionate number of heart events in the morning is what injures the heart during episodes of anger. I cannot minimize the importance of the relationship between the soul and body, where the soul's emotions can trigger a change in the body's chemical composition and harm us.

Several studies have examined this link. In the Determinants of Myocardial Infarction Onset Study, investigators interviewed more than sixteen hundred patients within one week of their heart attacks. They learned that 2.4 percent of these patients experienced an episode of anger within two hours preceding their attack. The most frequent source of their anger included arguments with family members (25 percent), problems at work (22 percent), and legal difficulties (8 percent).[6]

The Stockholm Heart Epidemiology Program reached similar conclusions about this connection. In interviews conducted with approximately seven hundred patients admitted to a coronary care unit, they found that people with an anger episode (described as "very angry") had a relative risk for a heart attack that increased ninefold over patients who were much calmer.[7]

I have listed just a few of the hundreds of scientific studies examining the link between anger—whether a chronic personality trait or sporadic outburst—and heart disease. I also reviewed the examples of Cain and Naaman, part of a long line of biblical instruction about anger. In the next section I will look at some proverbs that speak to anger and then conclude by examining specific conditions that can bear the seeds of bitterness. Unless we are vigilant in purging our souls of them, they will sprout and bring a ruinous harvest.

A Foolish Choice

Forsake foolishness and live.

—Proverbs 9:6

The Book of Proverbs is a wisdom-filled resource for learning about people. Not only does it describe all kinds and types, but it also gives advice on the best way to respond to them and how to behave around them. For instance, if you ever have the opportunity to visit a high-ranking government official, review Proverbs to learn the appropriate way to conduct yourself in his or her presence. If you are frustrated with office productivity, studying Proverbs might reveal the source of your problem is lazy people. Or if you aren't sure whether you or someone you know has anger issues, examine this book.

Proverbs uses the word *fool* to describe a person with uncontrolled, misdirected, and selfish anger. However, fools exhibit additional traits. Here are some that Proverbs describes:

- ♥ They are not inclined to listen to good advice: "The way of a fool is right in his own eyes, but he who heeds counsel is wise" (Proverbs 12:15).

- ♥ They resist repentance and blame others (or God) for their condition: "The foolishness of a man twists his way, and his heart frets against the Lord" (Proverbs 19:3).

- ♥ Conflict often appears in their relationships with their parents: "A wise son makes a glad father, but a foolish son is the grief of his mother" (Proverbs 10:1).

- ♥ Lacking humility, they think they are right all the time: "A fool has no delight in understanding, but in expressing his own heart" (Proverbs 18:2).

- ♥ Trying to discipline such a person is typically futile: "Though you grind a fool in a mortar with a pestle along with crushed grain, yet his foolishness will not depart from him" (Proverbs 27:22).

- ♥ They do not learn from past mistakes: "As a dog returns to his own vomit, so a fool repeats his folly" (Proverbs 26:11).

When we encounter fools, this last verse can help us recognize and accept the truth that we cannot change them. Only the Holy Spirit can transform a foolish temperament, so the most effective approach is prayer. However, keep this to yourself. If the object of your intercession learns about it, he or she may well take offense. (Such individuals don't believe they have any faults.) And when we identify a fool by one of the attributes I just listed, understand that their nature includes anger. Such foreknowledge can spare us grief by equipping us to respond appropriately when they manifest anger. Proverbs tells us exactly how to respond:

- ♥ Leave them alone: "Go from the presence of a foolish man, when you do not perceive in him the lips of knowledge" (Proverbs 14:7).

- ♥ Don't try to persuade them because it will only make things worse: "Do not speak in the hearing of a fool, for he will despise the wisdom of your words" (Proverbs 23:9).

♥ Accept that you will not reach a peaceful agreement: "If a wise man contends with a foolish man, whether the fool rages or laughs, there is no peace" (Proverbs 29:9).

♥ Understand that if you engage with such people long enough, you may be drawn into their behavior: "Do not answer a fool according to his folly, lest you also be like him" (Proverbs 26:4), and "A fool's lips enter into contention, and his mouth calls for blows" (Proverbs 18:6).

Since this final piece of advice is crucial, I listed two proverbs instead of one to emphasize the point. A fool's anger pulls like a magnet and can absorb like a sponge. It can draw us in, enticing us to yield to the flesh nature and respond in an ungodly manner. According to Proverbs 18:6, it even has the capacity to provoke us to the point of violence. For the sake of your heart, don't let that happen. Heed the warning of Proverbs 26:4 too. I often wonder how many wise people have suffered the consequences of angina, a heart attack, or sudden cardiac death because they allowed a fool to lure them into an argument and became angry themselves. Our best defense is to heed God's Word, refuse to verbally spar with anyone, swallow any pride, and humbly walk away from the situation. After all, the life you save might be your own!

The Roots of Bitterness

Search me, O God, and know my heart; try me, and know my anxieties; and see if there is any wicked way in me, and lead me in the way everlasting.

—PSALM 139:23–24

My husband entered the pastorate a few years after I completed my three-year residency in internal medicine. So I have been a pastor's wife for almost as long as I've been a board-certified physician. In these dual roles I have encountered and advised hundreds of men and women with deeply rooted anger. While the circumstances planting the seeds of anger are as unique and diverse as the people who struggle with it, I have observed that the underlying issue often falls into one of three categories.

A desire for vengeance

Cain's example shows how unchecked anger can lead to violence and even murder. However, when God punished Cain for killing his brother, Cain pleaded for mercy. The Lord responded with compassion. Cain feared for his life, believing someone would kill him in retaliation for murdering Abel. So God placed a mark on him and promised that "whoever kills Cain, vengeance shall be taken on him sevenfold" (Genesis 4:15). In doing so, God set the standard for retribution—it belongs to Him. He later decreed, "Vengeance is Mine" (Deuteronomy 32:35).

Yet, just a few generations later, Cain's descendant Lamech misrepresented what God did on behalf of Cain and assumed the role of avenger: "Then Lamech said to his wives: 'Adah and Zillah, hear my voice; wives of Lamech, listen to my speech! For I have killed a man for wounding me, even a young man for hurting me. If Cain shall be avenged sevenfold, then Lamech seventy-sevenfold" (Genesis 4:23–24). Offended by a young man, Lamech became the avenger. He took on the position that rightfully belongs to God, choosing to "get even" on his own terms. This wicked tendency is common among humans and goes hand in hand with anger.

Offenses are an inescapable part of life. However, when we are offended—and at some point we *will be*—it is vital that we guard our hearts against the tendency to respond in the spirit of Lamech or nurture a desire to retaliate. Often this desire can spring up whether another person offends us accidentally or deliberately, or even if the offender has asked for forgiveness. When our inner peace hinges on whether or not the offender suffers, anger has sprouted deep roots.

A problem with envy

Cain envied Abel because Abel's offering proved more pleasing to God. When Cain allowed his envy to go unchecked, it ultimately manifested itself as murderous anger. This speaks to the nature of envy—it defies any reasonable explanation. The person overtaken by envy behaves irrationally. The Bible describes it this way: "Wrath is cruel and anger a torrent, but who is able to stand before jealousy?" (Proverbs 27:4). We cannot stand against envy or its cousin, jealousy, because it defies logic. The logical mind asks, "Why didn't Cain simply make his own offering acceptable? Why wasn't Cain happy that his brother did well? What did Abel's relationship with God have to do with Cain in the first place?" While those questions are reasonable, the person consumed by envy loses the capacity for reason. Irrational, this individual proceeds to let anger take control. The consequences can prove deadly.

A sense of entitlement

Well aware of his position, power, and prestige, Naaman allowed arrogance to determine what was acceptable and unacceptable to him. Feeling entitled to special things and special treatment based on pride-driven self-assessment, he couldn't respond with humility. When the circumstances of life failed to meet his standard, he became angry.

Like the envious person, someone operating with a sense of entitlement can prove just as irrational. What did Elisha say to offend Naaman? Nothing. Elisha gave Naaman a clear-cut answer to his problem. What did Elisha do that harmed Naaman? Nothing. To the contrary, Elisha blessed him in a miraculous way. So why did Naaman respond with anger if Elisha neither said nor did anything offensive? Because the Syrian commander carried a preconceived notion of what he deserved. When Elisha did not fulfill his narcissistic expectations, he became the target of Naaman's anger. Pride blinded Naaman to reality—he was really entitled to leprosy. Since his anger distorted his impression of Elisha, he perceived the prophet as an offender rather than a source of healing.

Anger is detrimental to our physical, mental, and spiritual health. Left unchecked, it has the capacity to kill us, and it will certainly hinder our relationships. The first step to resolving anger is identifying it as a problem. Avoid the propensity to justify and rationalize anger, blame others, and avoid introspection. If this is your tendency, then make Psalm 139:23–24 part of your daily prayer and ask the Lord to reveal your heart. When He shows you the truth about your anger, don't become defensive. Agree with God that anger is a problem. In doing this, you will position yourself to receive His help to overcome. Your heart will thank you.

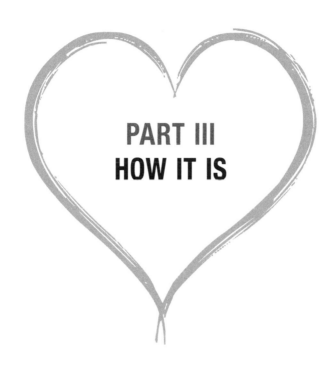

PART III
HOW IT IS

Chapter 8

EDEN IS OVER

So He drove out the man; and He placed cherubim at the east of the garden of Eden, and a flaming sword which turned every way, to guard the way to the tree of life.

Genesis 3:24

ONE OF THE HIGHEST COMPLIMENTS I RECEIVED ABOUT MY previous book, *Spiritual Secrets to Weight Loss*, came from a reader who told me that while it helped her lose a few pounds, she especially appreciated how it motivated her to study the Bible. Although a Christian for many years, she was unfamiliar with many of the passages of Scripture I referenced in that book. Taking a closer look at them encouraged her to become a more conscientious student of God's Word.

When writing to his young protégé, Timothy, Paul advised, "Be diligent to present yourself approved to God, a worker who does not need to be ashamed, rightly dividing the word of truth" (2 Timothy 2:15). Even though he addressed those words to a preacher, Paul's message applies to all Christians, whether we are in a leadership position or not. God commissioned each of us to diligently study the Bible. In doing so, we will benefit personally through spiritual growth while becoming better equipped to effectively use its precepts. This will instill a measure of confidence when we present the gospel to others or when we engage in dialogue about spiritual matters.

Today it is embarrassing that so many people who identify themselves as Christians lack even a basic understanding of the Bible. As a physician I must possess knowledge of the concepts and information in a medical textbook. Likewise, we who profess Christianity need to understand its "textbook." However, unlike in my professional life—where authorities can deny me licensing or board certification if I cannot demonstrate a reasonable level of medical knowledge—no such disciplinary measures exist for the Christian who lacks knowledge of the Word.

One area where many of us need to grow is in our comprehension of the first few chapters of Genesis, which describe God's creative process, including the creation of mankind. For many these stories are familiar—nearly every church member can quote, "In the beginning God created the heavens and the earth"—but our *understanding* must go beyond surface details. This is especially true regarding the account of Adam and Eve in the Garden of Eden. Many people learn this story as children, most often in Sunday school. Unfortunately, even after reaching adulthood many people maintain a childlike view of the first man and woman.

The *Illustrated Children's Bible Storybook* version covers about three pages. On page one an illustration shows Adam and Eve with smiling faces, standing in a beautiful garden on a bright, sunny day. It depicts them standing next to a bush with lush foliage and large, abundant leaves. A couple jut out to strategically cover the area between their waistlines and knees. The trees are studded with ripe fruit in bright shades of orange, red, and yellow. A few animals are close by, wearing smiles as cheerful as the humans. Eve's long, silky hair flows over each shoulder and extends down toward her midriff. It is a grand and glorious day in the Garden of Eden.

On page two the sun still shines brilliantly; everything remains plush and green. Only this day Eve's smile has faded, her countenance turned rather neutral. Her hair is still long and shimmering, with the leaves of a broad bush covering her waistline. However, on her other side is a tree. There a serpent with red, beady eyes and a menacing, ominous face winds down and around the trunk. As he speaks, it is easy to see that the snake's disturbing presence is the reason the brightness of her smile has withered.

Turn to page three. The sun has turned dark amid a gloomy horizon, as if a thunderstorm is approaching. Their smiles gone, Adam and Eve cower in fear. They look guilty, as if they are in big trouble. Those leaves that once jutted out around their waistlines? Gone. Though still long and silky, Eve's hair no longer flows over her shoulders. The once-innocent-looking couple now wears garments made of animal skin. They bear a striking resemblance to Tarzan and Jane.

Unfortunately many of us never progressed beyond this storybook level of understanding the events of Eden. In his first letter to the Corinthians Paul said, "When I was a child, I spoke as a child, I understood as a child, I thought as a child; but when I became a man, I put away childish things" (1 Corinthians 13:11). We too should put away childish things and mature in our understanding of the first few chapters of Genesis. Eden is over. When we comprehend this reality with adult insight, we will be better equipped to deal with life's challenges. And better motivated to take care of our bodies—including our hearts.

The "S" Word

For the wages of sin is death.

—ROMANS 6:23

Adam sinned. Eve sinned. Together they sinned. I need to emphasize this point because of its far-reaching ramifications. Sin changed everything and brought an end to perfect life on earth. Prior to their fall, the first man and woman enjoyed perfect bodies, perfect minds, a perfect environment, and a perfect relationship with God. The consequences of their mistake still haunt us. However, despite this reality, sin has become a dirty word in American's modern, "politically correct" culture.

In fact, when I started writing this section, I thanked the Lord for giving me the capacity to earn a living independent of writing. If I derived my livelihood from speaking and selling books, I would be tempted to avoid the topic of sin altogether. Many church leaders today rarely mention sin for fear of offending some within their congregations. Or they have bought into the mistaken notion that preaching against sin constitutes "judging." In addition to that, the decline in American church membership and concerns over attendance (and resulting contributions) can also influence messages from the pulpit. So can negative reactions from the pew, where church "cruisers" flock to pastors who proclaim everything is fine and God loves them, no matter what they do or how they act. Paul warned Timothy about this very thing: "For the time will come when they will not endure sound doctrine, but according to their own desires, because they have itching ears, they will heap up for themselves teachers; and they will turn their ears away from the truth, and be turned aside to fables" (2 Timothy 4:3–4).

Ironically, it is impossible to examine heart disease (or any disease, for that matter) from a Christian point of view without delving into this topic. While there was no disease in Eden, the garden vanished because of sin. From a biblical perspective, heart disease and sin are inextricably linked. Recognizing this connection is crucial not only in regard to physical disease but also to appreciate every aspect of life. There are dozens of things about the nature of sin we should understand as Christians. Here I will discuss two: (1) sin bears consequences, and (2) it affects others.

God provided Adam and Eve with everything they needed while issuing one restriction on their food: "And the LORD God commanded the man, saying, 'Of every tree of the garden you may freely eat; but of the tree of the knowledge of good and evil you shall not eat'" (Genesis 2:16–17). Did Adam and Eve have any concept of the consequences of their rebellion? When they yielded to temptation, did they realize how this would affect every generation to come? Although God warned them that "in the day that you eat of it you shall surely die" (verse 17), did they comprehend the full implications of disobedience?

Of course, we should not let fear of consequences be the reason we obey God. Adam and Eve should have done as they were told, regardless. Still, it is interesting to ponder whether they knew what would happen. The Bible isn't clear. We don't know if, in their perfect state and lacking any prior experience, they could grasp pain and suffering. Whatever the case, we see the end results—through original sin disease, disability, and death entered the world.

Sin's Impact

Not only does it bring consequences, but sin also affects others, including those who did not commit the sin. I am sure we can all recall doing or saying something that had a negative impact on someone else—a person not guilty of any transgression, often a loved one. Sin claims innocent victims. In the case of the original sin, all of mankind suffered because of Adam and Eve's decision, even though none of us were present in the Garden of Eden on that fateful day.

The consequences included death, which manifests itself in three forms:

- ♥ Spiritual death. We are born into this condition because of the "sin nature" passed down to us from Adam (Ephesians 2:1–2).

- ♥ Physical death. This is our "appointment" at the end of our lifetime: "And as it is appointed for men to die once, but after this the judgment" (Hebrews 9:27).

The only two exceptions were Enoch (Gen. 5:24) and Elijah (2 Kings 2:1–12), who were "translated" to heaven and did not experience physical death.

♥ Eternal death. Also called the "second death," this represents eternal separation from God.

We are born into spiritual death. Unless Christ returns first, we will keep our appointment with physical death. Yet through grace and faith in Christ, God spares us from eternal death. The second half of Romans 6:23, which opened this section, says, "But the gift of God is eternal life in Christ Jesus our Lord." This verse is not referencing physical life; it speaks of eternal life. Through God's grace we do not have to bear the eternal consequences of Adam and Eve's sin. This is a reason to rejoice!

Yet while we enjoy eternal life through accepting Jesus as Savior and Lord, we still must bear the consequences of physical disease, disability, and death. I have seen this reality confuse, frustrate, and cause despair among many Christians. Taking care of our bodies and optimizing our health will not nullify our Hebrews 9:27 appointment. Neither does the fact that God is able to miraculously heal disease. The vast majority of us will meet our end through disease rather than accident or calamity. Despite this reality, we can anticipate the day of restoration in the New Jerusalem, where "there shall be no more death, nor sorrow, nor crying. There shall be no more pain, for the former things have passed away" (Revelation 21:4). That day has not arrived. Until it does, we must accept that disability, disease, and death will remain in our midst.

I make this point because I so often witness confusion in this area. I have grieved with terminally ill patients who spent their last days overcome with guilt. They mistakenly believed (or their friends or families implied) that they were not steadfast in faith or otherwise they would have been healed. Instead of spending their final days in peace and reflecting on a lifetime of God's goodness, they harbored unwarranted fear, doubt, and even rejection. Instead of joyfully anticipating eternal life, they wondered why God refused to answer their prayer. Some desperately attempted "last ditch" efforts to increase their faith and receive miraculous healing. Yet what they hoped for didn't happen.

The same misunderstanding occurs among people with medical conditions that respond to lifestyle modifications. I always counsel patients that improving their diet, losing weight, and exercising regularly are necessary but may not eliminate their disease. Despite my caution, many set as an overriding goal getting off their medications. Sometimes, after extensive changes, their condition improves but disease remains. This is often when frustration surfaces: "Dr. Davis, what am I doing wrong? Why do I still need to take these pills?" I tell them how well they are doing and encourage them to keep up the good work. I also remind them that Eden is over, and although we should do all we can to optimize our health, God doesn't give any of us a disease-free guarantee.

When it comes to restoring health, please understand that I do not doubt God's capacity to perform miracles. I recognize Him as "Jehovah Rapha," our Healer. I understand the power of faith, that God responds to faith, and that sometimes He delivers people from diseases and near-death experiences. These are biblical truths. Yet the third chapter of Genesis also contains a biblical truth. Since the Bible does not contradict itself, we must be sure we are *complete* in our knowledge and grasp that the *consequences* of sin are not a reflection of God's lack of love. No matter how bad the consequences, when we experience them ("suffer" may be a better term), we should never assume God's love for us has diminished. It is profound and unconditional. However, all that He has done for us still doesn't spare us from the aftermath of original sin.

Cardiac Risk Factors

For since by man came death, by Man also came the resurrection of the dead. For as in Adam all die, even so in Christ all shall be made alive.

—1 CORINTHIANS 15:21–22

Although Eden has ended, Jesus brings us hope and restoration. By God's grace a time will come when what mankind lost through Adam will be restored through Christ. His grace is sufficient. Because of His grace we can take charge of the things we can change and live victoriously, in good health. Titus 2:12 teaches that by His grace we can deny worldly lusts and choose to live soberly. Sobriety does not refer exclusively to drunkenness; it also speaks to staying alert and attuning ourselves to spiritual matters. By His grace we can discipline our flesh and lead orderly lives. And by His grace we can know the fruit of the Spirit of self-control.

While those of us with risk factors for heart disease can change some, others we cannot. As I mentioned in the introduction, online tools can help estimate your ten-year risk for developing heart disease. In terms of risks, heart disease is more common in men. Prevalence increases with age; over the age of forty-five counts as a risk in men and over fifty-five for women. Heredity poses a higher risk too. In terms of family history, this is assessed by first-degree relatives—parents and siblings, not cousins, grandparents, or aunts and uncles. Obviously we can't change much about our gender, age, or family history. In addition, such risk is only statistically significant if cardiovascular disease appears at a relatively young age— namely, before age fifty-five in male relatives or sixty-five among female relatives.

Because it is much more common in men than in women, being male is an independent risk factor for heart disease. This is not to say that heart disease doesn't affect women; cardiovascular diseases are the number one cause of female death in the United States. Generally, heart disease diagnoses surface about ten years later among women. As women age, though, their risk becomes similar to that of men. Between approximately age forty-five and sixty-four one in nine women develops some form of cardiovascular disease. After age sixty-five this ratio climbs to one in three.[1]

The manifestations of heart disease in women may be quite different than in men. At one time, research studies of cardiovascular disease enrolled primarily white males. Physicians and other health care providers (including me) learned the "classic symptoms" of angina and myocardial infarction based on information gleaned from these single-dimensional trials. The health care community learned a valuable lesson about what can happen when we extrapolate data from a limited base. What is a "classic symptom" for white males may not be typical for females.

Women are more likely to use terms like "burning" or "sharp" to describe their heart pain; men often call it a "squeezing," "heaviness," or "tightness." Women are more likely to experience symptoms in places other than the chest (such as the neck, back, or throat), and they tend to have more symptoms unrelated to pain (i.e., nausea, weakness, fatigue, or shortness of breath). They are also more likely to experience angina from mental stress, not just physical exertion. Because of these differences, in the past women entering the emergency room with chest pains were typically treated less aggressively than men. They were *less* likely to receive cardiac monitoring, an evaluation by a cardiologist, or admission to a coronary care unit[2] but *more* likely to receive medications for anxiety.

Thankfully, as our knowledge about heart disease in women increases, these disparities are diminishing. However, this remains a real problem—doctors miss the diagnosis *less* often in women compared with times past, but they still miss it all too often. And women still receive less aggressive treatment than men, even as we progress through the second decade of the twenty-first century.

While risk factors of age, family history, and gender are beyond our ability to control, others can be modified. Through God's grace He equips us to live in a way whereby we can minimize the impact of these risk factors. We can change the way we live—not through willpower but through the equipping of the Holy Spirit. This is victorious living.

Earlier I discussed the impact of diet and exercise on dyslipidemia, hypertension, and type 2 diabetes. Each of these conditions has an undeniable genetic influence but is amenable to lifestyle modification. I will review each in more detail before concluding with a look at some environmental issues related to heart disease.

Dyslipidemia

The connection between dyslipidemia—in layman's terms, high cholesterol—and cardiovascular disease is well established. In chapter 1 I discussed the insights gained from the Framingham Heart Study. Another landmark study is the Multiple Risk Factor Intervention Trial (MRFIT).[3] The MRFIT table below shows the same consistent, continuous correlation between cholesterol levels and heart disease risk:[4]

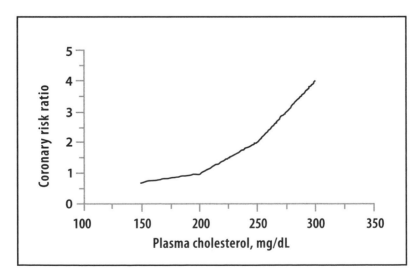

Based on such studies, medical authorities developed guidelines to help health care providers evaluate and treat dyslipidemia. Currently most physicians use the Third Report of the Expert Panel on Detection, Evaluation and Treatment of High Blood Cholesterol in Adults (ATP III) from the National Cholesterol Education Program (NCEP). At this writing, the fourth report is in the final stages of development. There will undoubtedly be some changes with ATP IV, so I encourage you to refer to the National Heart, Lung, and Blood Institute (www.nhlbi.nih.gov) to stay abreast of the latest recommendations.

The approach used by ATP III is based on LDL cholesterol, the presence or absence of other risk factors, and the presence or absence of preexisting coronary heart disease (or conditions that convey the same risk as coronary heart disease; I will discuss these "coronary heart disease equivalents" below). Physicians take all this information into account in determining the best approach to treatment and how aggressive that treatment should be.

Since LDL cholesterol is at the foundation of these guidelines, the first step is to obtain a blood sample while fasting to check your cholesterol profile. The U.S. Preventive Services Task Force and other expert groups have issued recommendations concerning the age at which lipid screening should begin. In men with no other risk factors for heart disease, that is thirty-five. The recommended age for screening women without risk factors is not as clear-cut; most guidelines recommend by age forty-five, while others suggest a younger age. Screening should start earlier (age twenty to thirty-five) if there are risk factors for heart disease, particularly obesity or a sedentary lifestyle.

The next step is determining whether you have any preexisting heart disease (e.g., angina or myocardial infarction) or a condition that places you in the same category as someone with heart disease. The latter are called "coronary heart disease equivalents" and include diabetes, peripheral vascular disease, carotid artery disease with symptoms, abdominal aortic aneurysm, or chronic kidney disease. If you have any of these conditions, then your doctor should assess your cholesterol goal *as if you have heart disease*— even if you have never exhibited a heart problem. This is why they are called "equivalents."

Keep in mind the approach to treating dyslipidemia is *individualized*. One key to determining the most appropriate treatment hinges on whether you fall into the category of "primary" or "secondary" prevention. If you don't have heart disease or an equivalent, or many risk factors, the aim in lowering cholesterol is primary prevention. The objective is to reduce the chance that you will ever have a primary heart event or first episode of disease. However, if you already have angina or other coronary artery disease, or been diagnosed with a heart disease equivalent, the goal is not primary prevention. Instead it is secondary prevention, whose aim is lowering the risk for subsequent heart problems. Secondary prevention features more aggressive treatment strategy and LDL cholesterol targets.

Once we know the LDL (or "bad") cholesterol level and if there are any preexisting heart disease or heart disease equivalents, the next step is evaluating for cardiac risk factors outside of cholesterol. These include hypertension, smoking, a family history of premature heart disease in a first-degree relative, and age (over forty-five for men and fifty-five for women). An HDL cholesterol level of less than 40 mg/dL counts as a risk, but if the HDL cholesterol is high (over 60 mg/dL), then it becomes a "negative" risk and removes a factor from the total count. In women, a low HDL is more predictive of heart disease risk than is a high LDL.[5] Armed with this data, a physician determines a goal for LDL cholesterol and whether lifestyle changes alone or in combination with medications can help a patient achieve this goal. This information is available in the ATP III guidelines, which can be accessed at http://www.nhlbi.nih.gov/guidelines/cholesterol/atp3full.pdf.

A preferred medication comes from the statin class, although other types can be used (especially if the body will not tolerate a statin; I will discuss this more in chapter 9). Considering everything I have reviewed, by now it should be obvious that everyone should strive to lead a healthier lifestyle. Maintaining a healthy body weight, exercising regularly, eating a nutritious diet, and breaking a tobacco habit will help lower LDL cholesterol and triglyceride levels and elevate good HDL cholesterol. Besides, quitting cigarettes will produce other health benefits.

Hypertension

Hypertension, or high blood pressure, affects about 30 percent of the adult population in the United States, or between 58 and 65 million people. Its prevalence has increased over time, paralleling our population's increased body weight.[6] As our population ages, experts expect these numbers to increase even further, since more than half of people over sixty-five suffer from high blood pressure. Currently about 12 percent of the population is over sixty-five, but by 2030 demographers forecast that it will reach 19 percent.[7]

Blood pressure readings consist of two numbers—the systolic pressure, the number on the top (listed first, i.e., "120 over 80"), and the diastolic pressure, the number on the bottom. The systolic blood pressure is the amount of pressure generated within the arteries when the heart contracts; the diastolic number is a measurement of the pressure generated when the heart relaxes. A committee of experts known as the Joint National Committee—or JNC—sets the guidelines for the diagnosis and treatment of hypertension. Every decade or so they release an updated set of guidelines. At this writing, the seventh set of guidelines (JNC-7) is in use, with a panel working on the eighth set (JNC-8).

The latest guidelines define a normal blood pressure as a systolic measurement of less than 120 millimeters of mercury (mmHg) *and* a diastolic measurement of less than 80 mmHg. Notice that *both* numbers must be within this range for a reading to be considered normal. "Prehypertension" is a systolic measurement of 120 to 139 *or* a diastolic measurement of 80 to 89. Hypertension is defined as a blood pressure greater than 140/90 and is divided into two stages:

♥ Stage 1: Systolic 140 to 159 mmHg *or* diastolic 90 to 99 mmHg

♥ Stage 2: Systolic more 160 mmHg *or* diastolic more than 100 mmHg

Hypertension is called the "silent disease" because it has no symptoms. Consequently many people with high blood pressure are unaware they have it. This speaks to the importance of regular medical checkups. Current guidelines for adults recommend screening at least every two years if the blood pressure is normal (less than 120/80) and at least annually for those with prehypertension.

Primary hypertension (also known as "essential" hypertension) is the most common type and accounts for as many as 95 percent of all cases.[8] Hypertension is labeled "secondary" when a doctor can identify a specific disease or disorder as the cause for blood pressure elevation. While the vast majority of hypertension is primary, there are certain clinical "red flags" that will prompt your physician to pursue the possibility of secondary hypertension. There are several risk factors and conditions associated with the development of essential hypertension:

♥ Race: Hypertension is more common and tends to be more severe among African Americans.

♥ Family history: The risk for developing hypertension increases if one or both parents have this condition.

♥ High dietary sodium and low dietary potassium: Sodium increases the blood pressure while potassium lowers it (more discussion of the roles of sodium and potassium in blood pressure appears in chapter 1).

- ♥ Obesity: Blood pressure increases with body weight. The rising blood pressure seen with aging is partially attributable to the tendency for people to gain weight as they grow older.

- ♥ Sedentary lifestyle: Regular exercise is beneficial for treating hypertension and can also delay or prevent its development.

- ♥ Excessive alcohol: Excessive alcohol use will increase blood pressure (more on this topic can be found in chapter 3).

- ♥ Personality: Hypertension may be more common in those whose personality traits include hostility and impatience.

- ♥ Dyslipidemia: Several studies have shown an association between high cholesterol and hypertension.[9]

- ♥ High-fructose corn syrup: Recent studies identify a connection between heavy consumption of high-fructose corn syrup and the development of hypertension.[10]

Like the risks for coronary artery disease, some risks for hypertension are unchangeable (e.g., race and family history) while we can modify others. It makes sense to adopt a lifestyle favorable to blood pressure, no matter what your measurement. Maintaining a healthy body weight, increasing exercise and physical activity, and following a diet high in potassium and low in sodium are feasible goals for everyone. These habits are especially important if your blood pressure is normal. Over time they will tilt the scales in your favor and protect you against developing hypertension as you age (or at least delay its onset).

Uncontrolled hypertension increases cardiovascular disease risk and affects other parts of the body, including the eyes and kidneys.

Chronic kidney disease is strongly associated with coronary artery disease and is considered an independent risk factor. About 80–85 percent of those with chronic kidney disease also have hypertension.

The risk of cardiovascular complications with hypertension increases with blood pressure: the higher the pressure, the higher the risk; the lower the pressure, the lower the risk. Recall the cardiovascular system is broad; its diseases include peripheral vascular disease and cerebrovascular disease (stroke) along with heart disease. All of these are more likely to occur with high blood pressure. This is why controlling blood pressure is vital, even if it requires multiple medications as well as lifestyle modifications. Unfortunately only about 34 percent of people with hypertension maintain a blood pressure below 140/90.[11] This means that the majority of people—even those taking medications—are not maintaining optimal control.

Type 2 Diabetes

Diabetes mellitus is a group of diseases characterized by high blood glucose (or sugar) levels. The body synthesizes insulin in the pancreas and functions as a glucose regulator. People with diabetes either do not make an adequate amount of this hormone, or their bodies are not sensitive to the insulin the pancreas produces. In general, the former describes type 1 diabetes, where the problem stems from *insulin deficiency*. The latter describes type 2 diabetes, where *insulin resistance* is the culprit—at least initially.

Since type 1 diabetics are insulin deficient, they cannot use oral medications but require insulin from the beginning of a diagnosis. Likewise, because insulin is necessary for survival, the disease is usually diagnosed soon after its onset. This is not the case with type 2 diabetes, where a prolonged period of time—even years—often passes between the onset of the disease and its diagnosis.

Type 2 diabetics initially have an adequate or even an excessive amount of insulin in the bloodstream. However, their bodies are not responding appropriately to the insulin that is circulating—hence the term "insulin resistance." Since insulin deficiency is not the problem, type 2 diabetics take oral medications. These either stimulate the pancreas to produce more insulin or "sensitize" the body to existing insulin. However, over time a type 2 diabetic's pancreas tends to "burn out," followed by a state of insulin deficiency. At this point (preferably much sooner) they need to start taking insulin.

Diabetes and prediabetes are diagnosed through blood tests. The fasting blood glucose and the hemoglobin A1c are the tests currently approved for screening. More elaborate tests are used in certain situations, such as pregnancy and for research. Your health care provider can determine when it is appropriate to begin screening and how often you should be screened—based on such variables as age, race, body weight, and other risk factors. If you are screened at a location other than a health care facility (for example, at a community health fair), it is crucial that you take those results to your physician, who can determine appropriate follow-up care.

Diabetes is common, affecting about 26 million Americans, according to 2011 estimates.[12] The vast majority is type 2—only 5–10 percent of diabetics are type 1.[13] In addition, about 79 million adults have "prediabetes," where blood glucose is too high but not high enough to meet the definition of diabetes.[14] Obviously people with prediabetes are at increased risk for developing diabetes, but they also have an increased risk for heart disease.

One of the most striking statistics is that 27 percent of people with diabetes (about 7 million Americans) do not know they have the disease.[15] This is due, in part, because symptoms are often easy to ignore. Excessive thirst or urination, weight loss, fatigue, irritability, excessive hunger, blurred vision, tingling in the toes and feet, and frequent infections are all signs of diabetes. Here I should emphasize the matter of weight loss. We all know how difficult it is to lose weight. If you ever find that losing weight has suddenly become easy, or that you are shedding pounds in spite of eating more, by all means get a screening. I have had many patients come to my office elated over finally losing weight, only to discover diabetes was the reason.

The number of people with diabetes and prediabetes increased significantly between 2008 and 2011. If current trends continue, the Centers for Disease Control and Prevention projects that one out of three American adults will have diabetes by 2050.[16] We urgently need to reverse these trends, especially for the sake of our children—who are developing type 2 diabetes with alarming frequency. As with heart disease, hypertension, and dyslipidemia, some risk factors for type 2 diabetes can be modified; some cannot. Risk factors include:

- ♥ Being overweight or obese
- ♥ Having prediabetes
- ♥ A family history of type 2 diabetes
- ♥ Age over forty-five
- ♥ A sedentary lifestyle
- ♥ Being a part of certain racial and ethnic groups (African Americans, Hispanic Americans, Asians, Pacific Islanders, Native Americans, and natives of Alaska all have increased risk.)
- ♥ High blood pressure, high triglyceride levels, or low HDL cholesterol
- ♥ Having diabetes during pregnancy, or giving birth to a baby weighing more than nine pounds

Obesity and overweight conditions are major risk factors for type 2 diabetes. So it is not surprising that the incidence and prevalence of diabetes has increased alongside increased BMI readings among adults and children. The two are so tightly linked that a doctor coined the term "diabesity" (and wrote a book about it) to reflect this connection. However, people can delay the development of type 2 diabetes or prevent it through lifestyle modifications, such as losing weight, improving the quality of the diet, and increasing physical activity. These lifestyle changes will benefit anyone, but are especially important when there are other, non-modifiable risks for diabetes like age, race, or family history.

Diabetes is a major risk factor for all forms of cardiovascular disease, but it carries other health risks too. Diabetes can affect the eyes with a complication called retinopathy. In addition, people with diabetes are more likely to develop glaucoma and cataracts. Diabetes can also damage the nerves and the kidneys. Still, there is good news. You can prevent (or least delay) complications through good diabetes control. This control is possible through various means—lifestyle modifications, oral medications, and medications administered by injection, including insulin. However, the latter aren't likely to work without the adoption of a healthy lifestyle, including a proper diet, adequate physical activity, and maintaining a healthy body weight. You can also reduce complications through regular follow-up appointments with your physician to obtain recommended screening tests, which can detect complications at an early stage.

The Environment

For we know that the whole creation groans and labors with birth pangs together until now.

—ROMANS 8:22

I have reviewed how disease, disability, and death resulted from original sin. Adam and Eve's sin didn't affect only humans and animals; it also affected the earth. In the third chapter of Genesis God confronted the serpent along with Adam and Eve and described the penalties for their disobedience. Of interest here is His statement to Adam: "Cursed is the ground for your sake; in toil you shall eat of it all the days of your life. Both thorns and thistles it shall bring forth for you" (Genesis 3:17–18). Where the land was once perfect, it is now imperfect. While still blessed by the land's provisions, we only see them through hard labor, and the earth harbors the potential to harm us. In recent years we have witnessed such destructive natural disasters as Hurricane Katrina; severe earthquakes in China, Haiti, and Japan; and tsunamis, mudslides, and floods across the world.

Just as God's children look forward to a time of restoration, so does the earth. Paul speaks to this in a passage in Romans 8, where he says that "creation itself also will be delivered from the bondage of corruption into the glorious liberty of the children of God" (verse 21). Paul personifies the earth in his description, saying it "groans and labors" in anticipation of its release one day from this curse.

Before original sin Adam served as the earth's caretaker, a task that remained his duty even after the Fall. The obligation to manage the earth passed on to his descendants and is now our responsibility. In many respects we fall short in the area of ecological stewardship. As a result, we live in an environment that can be toxic to our health. Air pollution is one manifestation of this potential for harm. Multiple studies over the past twenty years have confirmed what we previously knew intuitively: air pollution is a contributing factor to a variety of illnesses and even death.

Air pollution is a complex mixture of gases, liquids, and particles. The particle component includes black carbon, metals, nitrates, and sulfates, along with other by-products of combustion. Some pollutants are emitted "naturally," coming from such sources as volcanic eruptions and forest fires. However, many other pollutants are man-made. They enter the atmosphere through vehicle emissions, industry, and power plants. Both are harmful. Fine particulate matter is made up of particles less than 2.5μm (a μm measures a millionth of a meter) in diameter. These size particles play a major role in causing or exacerbating disease.

While respiratory illnesses are certainly connected to air pollution, air pollution also plays a role in an increased risk for cardiovascular disease. In 2004 the American Heart Association (AHA) released a report on air pollution and cardiovascular disease in which it confirmed the increased risk to the heart from short-term and long-term exposure to air pollution, specifically fine particulate matter. The report listed possible ways in which this happens, including chronic inflammation, constriction of the arteries, or enhancing the body's propensity to form blood clots.[17]

In 2010 the AHA issued an updated report, which included data from studies conducted in the interim. Researchers reached the following conclusions:

- ♥ Exposure to fine particulate matter, ranging from a few hours to weeks, can trigger cardiovascular disease-related mortality and nonfatal cardiovascular events.

- ♥ Long-term exposure (years) increases the risk of death from cardiovascular disease to a greater extent than short-term exposure.

- ♥ In segments of the population with long-term high exposure, life expectancy is reduced by several months to a few years.

- ♥ Reducing the level of fine particulate matter is associated with a decrease in cardiovascular mortality within as short a span as a few years.

In their latest statement these experts wrote, "It is the opinion of the writing group that the overall evidence is consistent with a causal relationship between PM2.5 [fine particulate matter] exposure and cardiovascular morbidity and mortality. This body of evidence has grown and been strengthened substantially since the first American Heart Association scientific statement was published [in 2004]. Finally, PM2.5 exposure is deemed a modifiable factor that contributes to cardiovascular morbidity and mortality."[18]

I believe there is good news and bad news here. The bad—the proven association between air pollution and heart disease (not to mention its association with other diseases). However, the good news is that the experts have categorized air pollution as a "modifiable factor." This means we can do something about it. It may not be easy or convenient, but it is possible. All it takes is a little commitment, consistency, and resolve, which happen to be the same character traits required to change other "modifiable factors." Just as we can choose a diet beneficial to our hearts and exercise regularly to strengthen them, so we can "go green" to protect them. In doing so, not only do we glorify God by taking care of His temple, but we also honor Him by becoming better stewards of the earth He entrusted to us.

Chapter 9

MEDICATIONS AND PROCEDURES

Along the bank of the river, on this side and that, will grow all kinds of trees used for food; their leaves will not wither, and their fruit will not fail. They will bear fruit every month, because their water flows from the sanctuary. Their fruit will be for food, and their leaves for medicine.

Ezekiel 47:12

R EMARKABLE AND AWE-INSPIRING, VISIONS FROM GOD PRO- vide the kind of hope that we cannot find from focusing on human strengths or accomplishments. This is why John's vision of the New Jerusalem coming down from heaven in Revelation 21:1–2 still inspires believers across the world nearly two thousand years after he wrote those prophetic words. Though not as familiar, but no less startling, is the vision Ezekiel received about the restoration of Jerusalem. When he penned his prophecy, the city lay in ruins.

The above verse appears in the passage about this vision. As a young man, Ezekiel had been taken captive by the Babylonian Empire. In Babylon he served as both priest (his inherited duty) and prophet (God's calling). Ezekiel opened his book with prophecies concerning Jerusalem's destruction, followed by chapters about God's judgment of surrounding nations. In the final segment that I reference above, God gives Ezekiel a glimpse of Israel in the distant future, during the millennial period of Christ's reign.

Ezekiel saw a stream flowing from under the temple in Jerusalem and progressively widening and deepening into a great river. This river flowed into the Dead Sea, converting it from a place of death to one of life. Its "dead" name originates with this sea's high salt content—six times greater than the oceans and too concentrated to sustain life. However, this new river transformed it into a sea teeming with fish and vegetation, as well as supplying fresh water to multiple, fruit-bearing trees on shore, their leaves containing medicinal properties.

Since this kind of metamorphosis is humanly impossible, believing God can transform a dead body of water into a source of life and healing requires more than a shallow faith. However, that isn't the only reason for this vision's significance. Ezekiel 47:1–12 is just one of many biblical passages that I believe counter the negative reputation medications have garnered in recent years. Granted, our primary objective in maintaining good health is to live in ways that edify the body naturally. Yet, as I discussed in chapter 8, we cannot ignore the reality of disease, disability, and death in a fallen world. Sometimes, despite our best efforts to adhere to a healthy lifestyle, we need medications and medical procedures.

In this chapter I will examine several heart-healthy prescriptions, dietary supplements, vitamins, and minerals. Among the drugs I will review are those used to control hypertension and high cholesterol, since they are classified as cardiovascular medications. Tobacco is a major risk factor for heart disease, but the prescription and over-the-counter drugs available to help people quit are not cardiovascular medications per se, so I will not discuss them. Likewise, the medications used to treat type 2 diabetes are not for the heart, even though heart disease is the main complication of diabetes. I will, however, briefly review some facts on two categories of diabetes medications that show that they may actually increase (rather than reduce) the risk for cardiovascular disease. I will conclude with an overview of some procedures for treating coronary artery disease.

Medications

> No longer drink water exclusively, but use a little wine for the
> sake of your stomach and your frequent ailments.
> —1 TIMOTHY 5:23, NAS

Timothy was Paul's friend, disciple, "son" in ministry, and a pastor of the church in Ephesus. Paul wrote his protégé two letters of encouragement and instruction, advising him how to lead his congregation. In the above verse Paul suggested a way of addressing his own needs. Though the Bible doesn't indicate the nature of Timothy's "frequent ailments," we can surmise from the rest of Paul's letter that whatever troubled Timothy physically was likely exacerbated by the pressure that comes with church leadership. As the wife of a pastor, I am keenly aware of the burdens confronting these leaders. While opposition from sources outside the church is to be expected, in my opinion the strains originating with believers on the inside are more detrimental.

While writing this manuscript, heart attacks claimed the lives of five pastoral friends or acquaintances of my husband; all were under the age of sixty. I am not suggesting that their congregations were in any way culpable. While I don't blame anyone for these sorts of tragedies or other stress-related illnesses that afflict pastors, I must emphasize a point made by the author of Hebrews, who admonished us to undergird church leaders: "Obey your leaders and submit to their authority. They keep watch over you as men who must give an account. Obey them so that their work will be a joy, not a burden, for that would be of no advantage to you" (Hebrews 13:17, NIV). A pastor's congregation should be a peace-filled fellowship, a source of joy and strength, refreshing and not distressing.

We will be blessed when we purpose in *our* hearts to make *our pastor's* heart happy!

Pastors have a responsibility also to guard their hearts by taking proactive steps to protect their health, whether through improving their diet, getting more rest, or keeping a better balance between their personal and work lives. Timothy is an example of proactive steps to meet physical needs. Granted, just as we don't know Timothy's specific ailments, neither do we know how he responded to Paul's recommendation. However, given Paul's authority and Timothy's high regard for his mentor, I cannot imagine Timothy ignoring it. I suspect Timothy paid more attention to his *total* well-being—spirit, mind, and body. Whether church leaders or members, we all face "frequent ailments" (diseases) and must pursue the best options for our health, even if that means taking medications.

Prescription and Over-the-Counter Medications for Hypertension

Several different types effectively treat hypertension. Some medications do more than lower blood pressure, also improving or restoring heart functions for someone with congestive heart failure, or improving the odds of survival after a myocardial infarction. However, although these medications will all lower blood pressure, the degree varies from drug to drug and person to person. Choices are influenced by many variables, including:

- ♥ Age (younger people may respond better to some medications than older people)

- ♥ The presence of other conditions (e.g., heart failure, diabetes, kidney disease)

- ♥ Race (for example, African Americans are especially responsive to diuretics)

♥ Gender (younger women considering pregnancy should not use certain drugs, particularly ACE inhibitors)

♥ Cost (generics vs. brand names, and whether the medication is available under a particular insurance plan)

More than likely, the greatest benefit with respect to heart disease and mortality comes purely from bringing the numbers down—irrespective of the agent selected. Still, there are unique advantages to one drug (or category of drugs) over another. I will not provide a review of major clinical trials evaluating blood pressure medications, even though they are important and their results help guide health care providers in selecting the appropriate drug for a given patient. Rather than an exhaustive review, the following table lists the major categories and properties worth noting. Additional information on hypertension appears in chapter 8.

Category	Examples	Properties
Angiotensin-converting enzyme (ACE) inhibitors	benazepril, captopril, enalapril, fosinopril, lisinopril, moexipril, perindopril, quinapril, ramipril, trandolapril	This class is the first choice for people who have had a heart attack, people with heart failure or dysfunction of the heart's left ventricle, people with diabetes, or people with chronic kidney disease.
Angiotensin II receptor blockers (ARB)	candesartan, eprosartan, irbesartan, losartan, olmesartan, telmisartan, valsartan	The benefits are essentially the same as those with ACE inhibitors.

Category	Examples	Properties
β-blockers and α/β blockers	*Beta-blockers:* acebutolol, atenolol, betaxolol, bisoprolol, carteolol, metoprolol, nadolol, nebivolol, penbutolol, pindolol, propranolol, timolol *Alpha/beta blockers:* carvedilol, labetalol	β-blockers improve survival after a myocardial infarction and should ideally be started within twenty-four hours of a heart attack. In the absence of contraindications, anyone who has had a heart attack should continue them indefinitely. With respect to hypertension in the *absence* of a previous heart attack, β-blockers are generally not recommended as single, first-line therapy but are reserved as add-on therapy.
Calcium antagonists	*Dihydropyridines:* amlodipine, felodipine, isradipine, nicardipine, nisoldipine, nifedipine *Non-dihydropyridines:* diltiazem, verapamil	Calcium antagonists (calcium "channel blockers") can be used as initial or add-on therapy.
Diuretics	*Thiazides:* hydrochlorothiazide, chlorothiazide, chlorthalidone, indapamide *Aldosterone antagonists:* spirono-lactone, eplerenone *Loop diuretics:* furosemide, bumetanide, torsemide, ethacrynic acid *Potassium sparing:* triamterene, amiloride *Multiple sites of action:* meto-lazone	Thiazide diuretics can be used as initial therapy or add-on therapy. They are particularly beneficial when fluid accumulation is a problem; for example, in people with heart failure or kidney disease.

Category	Examples	Properties
Central α-agonists and vasodilators	*Central alpha-agonists:* methyldopa, clonidine, guanabenz, guanfacine *Vasodilators:* hydralazine, minoxidil	Central alpha-agonists and vasodilators are not prescribed as initial therapy but are reserved for people with resistant hypertension, which is defined as blood pressure that remains uncontrolled despite the use of three different types of medicines, including a diuretic. In patients with congestive heart failure whose symptoms persist despite optimal therapy, the addition of hydralazine in combination with a nitrate is beneficial, especially in African Americans.
α-adrenergic blockers	prazosin, doxazosin, terazosin, phenoxybenzamine	Alpha-adrenergic blockers are not recommended as initial single therapy but are used as add-on therapy. They may be particularly beneficial in older men who have urinary symptoms as a result of enlargement of the prostate gland, as they help to improve emptying the bladder.
Direct renin inhibitor	aliskiren	This is the most recent class of medications developed. Aliskiren was approved by the FDA in 2007, and at this writing remains the only medication in this class. Its role in managing hypertension (i.e., first-line or add-on therapy) remains unclear until further studies become available.

In addition to the single medications listed in the table, many come in combinations of two to four drugs in a single pill, boosting the available options to more than two hundred. Nearly everyone with hypertension can find a convenient regimen, one easily tolerated and with few or no side effects. However, despite these advances, an alarming number of people with hypertension still show poorly controlled blood pressure. The Centers for Disease Control and Prevention (CDC) estimates that from 2005 to 2008 only 46 percent of the 68 million people with hypertension had achieved optimal control, even though they had been prescribed medications.[1]

Lipid-Lowering Agents

Statins

These include atorvastatin, fluvastatin, lovastatin, pitavastatin, pravastatin, rosuvastatin, and simvastatin. Statins are the most widely prescribed of medications used to treat high cholesterol. They are highly effective at lowering bad LDL cholesterol, with two decades of research confirming that they decrease the risk for such cardiovascular events as heart attack and stroke, both among people with heart disease and those without any known problems. In an analysis of more than ninety thousand patients, findings showed that for every 39 mg/dL that statins lower LDL cholesterol level, the risk for a major cardiac event is reduced by 25 percent.[2]

Statins don't often produce side effects, but all have the potential to cause muscle damage (myopathy); some have a greater tendency than others. People taking statins should let their physician know if they develop muscle pain or weakness so that he or she can determine whether this stems from a medication side effect.

Non-statin cholesterol-lowering drugs

These non-statins include fibric acid derivatives (gemfibrozil, fenofibrate), bile acid sequestrants (cholestyramine, colestipol, colesevelam), nicotinic acid (niacin), and ezetimibe.

Lowering LDL cholesterol with statins will reduce the chance of heart attack and stroke among people with risk factors for cardiovascular disease. However, LDL cholesterol is not the only lipid affecting coronary arteries. Both a low HDL cholesterol level (less than 40 mg/dL in men and less than 50 mg/dL in women) and a high triglyceride level (more than 200 mg/dL) are associated with increased risk for cardiovascular disease. Several non-statin cholesterol-lowering medications improve HDL and triglycerides, along with lowering LDL.

Unlike statins, though, the clinical benefits of these medications are not as firmly established. While large studies have confirmed that statin-mediated lowering of LDL translates into fewer heart attacks and strokes, no similarly strong evidence exists for non-statin drugs. In other words, a medication may make the numbers look good, but the most important measurements are clinical outcomes. Namely, are there fewer cardiovascular events—such as heart attack and stroke—that accompany those numbers? In the future, as more randomized clinical trials occur, we will obtain much needed information on whether non-statins improve the risk for cardiovascular disease.

I would add, though, that if your physician has prescribed a non-statin, by all means take it! They are used commonly; sometimes I prescribe them. Still, I believe consumers should be aware of the data regarding clinical outcomes and the presence or absence of evidence relating to improved cardiovascular risk so they can use this knowledge in making decisions about their medications.

Anti-Platelet Agents

When an atherosclerotic plaque ruptures, it releases substances that activate platelets. These platelets become "sticky" and clump together to form the core of the clot that goes on to block a heart artery. Anti-platelet medications are especially important in the management of unstable angina and myocardial infarction. They are also necessary in preventing re-blockage after the artery's opening by means of a percutaneous coronary intervention (or PCI, which I will discuss later).

Aspirin is the most common anti-platelet agent and is effective at doses lower than those typically used for pain relief. In addition to use in acute coronary events, aspirin also is effective in preventing a heart attack and stroke in people who have never had a cardiovascular event (primary prevention) and reducing the chance of a recurrent heart attack or stroke in people who have had such an event (secondary prevention).

Other oral anti-platelet medications are not used for primary prevention but may be prescribed after a coronary event occurs or after a cardiovascular procedure (such as insertion of a heart stent). These generally are taken along with aspirin and include dipyridamole, clopidogrel, ticlopidine, ticagrelor, and prasugrel.

Type 2 Diabetes Medications

Several medications are available for treating type 2 diabetes. Some are taken by mouth, others are given by injection, but all should be used in conjunction with lifestyle modification—a heart-healthy diet, regular exercise, and weight loss when indicated. The main goal for good diabetes control is to reduce complications, especially damage to the kidneys (nephropathy), nerves (neuropathy), and eyes (retinopathy). While all of the available medications are able to improve the glucose and hemoglobin A1c levels, as we discussed in the section on non-statin cholesterol-lowering medications, the main objective is not numbers but outcomes. In other words, do people taking the medication experience fewer complications in the long term, or do they just have nice looking laboratory values?

The thiazolidinediones (TZDs) are one category of medications used to treat type 2 diabetes. At this writing, two are available in the United States: rosiglitazone and pioglitazone. The TZDs have been shown to improve not only glucose control but also the cholesterol profile and several markers of inflammation. Based on this, one might assume they would be the ideal medication for people with diabetes. But it turns out that long-term data do not show any significant reduction in cardiovascular complications in people taking TZDs. To the contrary, the TZDs have a tendency to cause fluid retention and can actually increase the risk of heart failure.[3]

Another very popular category of drugs used to treat type 2 diabetes is the sulfonylureas. These medications have been used for decades, and while they will definitely improve the glucose and hemoglobin A1c levels, there is not much data on whether they actually lower the risk for cardiovascular disease in the long run. Interestingly a 2012 study published in the *Annals of Internal Medicine* found that, compared to the drug metformin, people started on sulfonylureas had a higher chance of having a heart attack or stroke.[4]

For now, both categories remain on the market with FDA approval. I am not suggesting that anyone currently prescribed these drugs should stop taking them. But, as in all things, discuss their use with your health care provider, and let the data I've presented serve to motivate you to maximize the "tried and true" benefits found in lifestyle modification.

Vitamins, Minerals, and Dietary Supplements

Antioxidant vitamins include A (beta-carotene), C (ascorbic acid), and E (alpha-tocopherol). There are many steps in the process of going from "clean" arteries to the plaques, blockages, and dysfunctions that characterize cardiovascular disease. If it were a recipe, atherosclerosis would contain a long list of ingredients and an elaborate set of directions. One ingredient would be oxidation, a key component in the initiation and progression of coronary artery disease.

Normal metabolism involves oxidation, a process that generates molecules known as peroxides and oxygen-free radicals. These highly reactive molecules damage the body's tissues and proteins, which contributes to atherosclerosis. Oxidized LDL cholesterol and oxidation of the endothelial cells in the blood vessels play a role in this; they are a factor in other diseases, such as cancer and the process of aging.

Under normal circumstances the free radicals formed as a by-product of metabolism are kept under control through an efficient system designed to neutralize them. Antioxidants are like a "cleanup crew." These scavenger molecules target free radicals and "deactivate" them, which defuses their damaging effects. Our bodies produce antioxidants in the form of enzymes, but they also come through our diet via foods containing beta-carotene (vitamin A), ascorbic acid (vitamin C), and alpha-tocopherol (vitamin E), the three major antioxidant vitamins.

There is a definite association between a diet rich in antioxidant vitamins and a lower risk for heart disease, as indicated by multiple observational studies. However, such studies have several limitations, including the fact they do not necessarily establish cause and effect, which can mislead anyone unfamiliar with statistical analysis. Another problem with observational studies of dietary antioxidant vitamins is they do not tease out other possibilities that might contribute to the findings. In other words, are there additional compounds in fruits and vegetables that have a heart-protective effect or enhance the effect of the vitamin? Are people who eat a vitamin-rich diet also engaging in other heart-healthy activities? Do such individuals consume a smaller proportion of foods detrimental to the heart? Could it be their diet correlates to a lower BMI, which strongly influences cardiovascular risk?

These sorts of questions are important to consider. With respect to antioxidant vitamins, randomized trials show different results than observational studies. Briefly, observational studies are just that—they make observations on a group of individuals in the absence of an intervention. But in randomized trials, the "gold standard" of research, participants are randomly assigned to groups, either to receive the intervention or not, and followed over extended periods of time. Studies examining the use of antioxidant vitamin supplements for the prevention of heart disease have not shown positive results. To the contrary, most show no effect; some demonstrate harm.

In the Finnish Alpha-Tocopherol Beta-Carotene Cancer Prevention Study and the Physician's Health Study, men taking beta-carotene had a higher incidence of death from heart disease.[5] In addition, multiple studies have shown a greater rate of death from all causes in people taking high doses of vitamin E.[6] So, while observational studies point to a benefit from a diet rich in antioxidant vitamins, randomized trials reveal there are additional questions to be answered and that there is more to the equation than vitamins. The same statement applies to folic acid and B-complex vitamins.

Folic acid and B-complex vitamins

Amino acids are the building blocks for proteins. While we get amino acids through diet, our bodies are able to convert some amino acids into others. In the step-by-step conversion of the amino acid methionine into cysteine, we produce an intermediate product known as homocysteine. High levels of homocysteine are associated with an increased risk for heart disease. Some people have too much homocysteine because of a genetic disorder where they are deficient in the enzymes necessary to complete the conversion. However, homocysteine commonly accumulates as a result of nutritional deficiencies, specifically from inadequate dietary folate and vitamins B_6 and vitamin B_{12}.

Since taking folic acid (the synthetic form of folate) and B-vitamin supplements will definitely lower homocysteine levels, one might intuitively conclude that they should also reduce the risk for heart disease. However, just as with the findings with antioxidants, several medical studies have demonstrated this is not so. The HOPE-2 clinical trial examined more than five thousand adults with cardiovascular disease or diabetes. Researchers gave participants either vitamin supplements to lower their homocysteine levels or a placebo. While homocysteine dropped among supplement users (and increased in those on the placebo), the two groups showed no difference in the rate of heart attack, stroke, or death from cardiovascular disease.[7]

Not surprisingly, then, current data does not support the use of vitamins for prevention or treatment of cardiovascular disease. This doesn't mean we should avoid vitamins, but we must understand that they cannot replace a heart-healthy diet containing natural, nutrient-rich foods, including antioxidants and B vitamins. Likewise, vitamins will not undo the detrimental effects of a poor diet. Since they won't reverse the consequences of unhealthy habits, they also don't represent a license to forsake a prudent, heart-healthy lifestyle.

Calcium

Calcium is necessary for healthy bones. Though vital at every age, this mineral is especially important for women after menopause, when the rate of bone loss accelerates. Calcium and vitamin D are recommended for the prevention and treatment of osteoporosis, along with such measures as smoking cessation and exercise.

As with most nutrients, the ideal sources of calcium come from food. However, since many people can't tolerate dairy products—the most abundant source of calcium—they must turn to supplements.

The effects of calcium supplements on the risk of cardiovascular disease is a source of controversy. While some studies show these supplements produce a small decrease in blood pressure and improvement in HDL cholesterol levels, they haven't demonstrated a lowering of the incidence of heart disease. For instance, in the Women's Health Initiative trial, calcium and vitamin D supplementation had no effect on the rate of heart attack or stroke in a group of thirty-six thousand postmenopausal women over a period of seven years.[8] Two more recent analyses raised some concerns that calcium supplements may *increase* the risk for heart attack and stroke.[9]

The jury is still out on whether this is indeed the case, since analyses like these do not necessarily prove cause and effect and are fraught with other limitations. Additional randomized controlled trials are warranted to clarify their findings. Until such studies are done, the best recommendation is taking combined calcium and vitamin D supplements, with total calcium (dietary and supplemental) not exceeding 2,000 mg per day.

Fish oil (n-3 fatty acids)

More than fifty years ago reports surfaced about the low prevalence of heart disease among Greenland's Eskimos (Inuits). Now we know the reason for this was related to their diet, composed primarily of whale and seal. These meats are rich in omega-3 (n-3) fatty acids. Along with a "heart-healthy" lipid profile, studies of the Inuits show they have reduced platelet activity and a lower incidence of immune and inflammatory diseases.

As I mentioned in chapter 1, polyunsaturated fats have a chemical structure made up of more than one double bond ("poly" meaning "many"). These fats are named according to the number of double bonds, configuration, and position on the fat chain. The n-6 and n-3 fatty acids—linoleic acid and alpha-linolenic acid (ALA), respectively—are essential nutrients for mammals. Our bodies lack the enzymes needed to synthesize them. Walnuts and plant oils are good sources for both, especially soybean, flaxseed, linseed, and canola oils. Humans are able to convert linoleic acid and ALA ingested from plants into eicosapentaenoic acid (EPA) and docosahexaenoic acid (DHA), the n-3 fatty acids most relevant in protecting the heart. However, this conversion from plant oils and nuts is fairly limited. Consequently, the main dietary source of n-3 fatty acid is not from plants but fish, especially oily varieties like salmon, mackerel, trout, herring, and sardines.

After observation of Greenland's Eskimos, subsequent studies of other populations showed the same protective effects from diets rich in omega oils. There is a clear, well-documented inverse association between fish consumption and heart disease. As the amount of fish in the diet *increases*, the risk of cardiovascular disease *decreases*.

Fish oil has several beneficial effects on the heart. It improves the lipid profile by lowering triglycerides and increasing HDL cholesterol. It lowers the heart rate and blood pressure and helps blood vessels and the heart muscle to relax. Because of these findings, the American Heart Association (AHA) recommends adults eat fish at least twice a week, along with vegetables and vegetable oils high in ALA. It also advises men and women known to have cardiovascular disease consume approximately 1 gram daily of combined EPA and DHA in the form of fish or fish oil supplements.

Fish oil supplements are convenient, especially for people who aren't accustomed to eating fish on a regular basis. Supplements also have the advantage of being free of contaminants such as mercury, which has been detected in some species of fish. But the benefits associated with *dietary* sources of fish oil may not be found in *supplemental* sources. A 2012 review and meta-analysis published in the *Journal of the American Medical Association* failed to show any benefit from fish oil supplements with respect to myocardial infarction, stroke, sudden cardiac death, or death from any cause.[10]

Undoubtedly further studies will be done to confirm these findings. For now, the American Heart Association's recommendations still stand with regard to taking supplements, but (as in all things) the natural source appears to hold the benefits.

Soy

Soy foods and food products (e.g., tofu, endamame, soy burgers, and soy butter) are excellent sources of protein. Like other plant-derived proteins, they do not come "packaged" with the saturated fat found in animal-based proteins. In and of itself, this qualifies them as a heart-healthy food. However, some in the fields of health and nutrition promote soy's cardiovascular benefits beyond these properties. Unlike fish oil, where observational studies and randomized trials confirm its cardiovascular benefits, the evidence for soy is weaker.

Early studies with soy suggested an improvement in cholesterol, but subsequent reviews concluded that any unique heart benefits were insignificant. One found that consuming large amounts of soy—in quantities representing approximately half of protein intake—decreased LDL cholesterol by only 3 percent. The study also showed no effect on HDL cholesterol, triglycerides, lipoprotein (a), or blood pressure.[11] Because of the absence of clinical evidence, the AHA does not recommend soy supplements for cardiovascular protection. Still, available data indicates health benefits in line with plant-based foods: they are high in polyunsaturated fats, vitamins, minerals, and fiber, and they are low in saturated fats.

Red yeast rice

A fermented rice product, red yeast rice is used in Chinese cooking and as a medicinal agent. It contains varying amounts of monacolins, which are naturally occurring substances that have an effect similar to statins. Some rather small studies have confirmed a significant drop in LDL cholesterol with red yeast rice. One study of some 60 patients who could not tolerate statins because of muscle pain showed they didn't experience pain when taking red yeast rice.[12]

While promising, presently there are no long-term studies to evaluate safety and whether red yeast rice lowers cardiovascular outcomes, such as heart attack and stroke. In addition, as with other dietary supplements, the amount of active ingredient may vary from brand to brand, which affects their efficacy.

Plant sterols

Plant sterols have a chemical structure similar to that of cholesterol and are thought to work by blocking the absorption of cholesterol in the intestines. Available in dietary supplements, several foods contain plant sterols, including margarine, orange juice, and rice milk. Studies have shown that these foods reduce serum cholesterol. To date, however, no studies demonstrate that they lower the risk for coronary heart disease, nor do any confirm the safety of long-term use. One animal study found detrimental effects in the blood vessels of mice taking a diet supplemented with plant sterols, with an increased rate of atherosclerosis and impaired endothelial function.[13]

Until further research demonstrates safety and a reduction in the risk for cardiovascular disease, the American Heart Association advises against routine use by most people of foods containing plant sterols. It recommends use be reserved for adults who require LDL cholesterol reduction because of a known history of cardiovascular disease, or if people are at high risk for its development.

Flavonoids

Certain fruits and vegetables are rich in a class of substances known as flavonoids, which are chemicals that have attracted considerable attention because of their effects on the cardiovascular system and cardiovascular risk factors. While most fruits and vegetables should be part of a heart-healthy diet, those with high concentrations of flavonol are particularly beneficial. In the Iowa Women's Health Study, investigators followed nearly thirty-five thousand women for sixteen years and found a lower risk of death from heart disease among females with a higher consumption of flavonoid-rich foods.[14]

While I will limit my following discussions to tea and cocoa, the table below lists some common foods and beverages high in flavonol, along with their concentrations.

Food or Beverage	Flavonol Content (mg/kg or mg/L)
Cocoa	460–612
Beans	350–550
Apricots	100–250
Cherries	50–220
Peaches	50–140
Blackberries	130
Apples	20–120
Black tea	60–500
Green tea	100–800
Red wine	80–300

Tea

A large, population based study in Japan found that the higher green tea consumption, the lower the risk of death from cardiovascular disease.[15] While all of tea's heart protective effects are not clear, it does lower total and LDL cholesterol levels, which is one possible mechanism. In animal studies, tea showed reduced absorption of cholesterol from the intestines, reduced the amount of cholesterol produced by the liver, and increased the amount of cholesterol excreted in the feces.

Green teas represent a rich source of flavonoids, while black tea contains theaflavin, a product derived from the fermentation of green tea to form black tea. Both have favorable effects on cholesterol levels. In one study involving 240 men and women with high cholesterol—and who were already on a diet low in saturated fat—participants who took theaflavin-enriched green tea extract experienced a significant drop in LDL cholesterol levels, compared to those who took a placebo.[16]

While tea should not replace a statin in people with high risk for heart disease, it can be used in addition to one. For men and women at low risk for heart disease, but who have mild to moderately elevated cholesterol, green tea is worth trying in conjunction with diet modification.

Cocoa

Cocoa exhibits effects similar to those of tea on the cholesterol profile, with a reduction in LDL cholesterol and elevation of the good HDL. In addition, cocoa contains a blood-pressure-lowering effect and may decrease insulin resistance. However, keep in mind that there is a big difference between natural cocoa and milk chocolate. The latter is a combination of cocoa, sugar, milk, and other ingredients that can contribute to weight gain, which will presumably increase cardiovascular risk. I qualify that statement with "presumably" because at least one meta-analysis of several observational studies found a reduced rate of cardiac and metabolic diseases (including stroke) in people who had a higher consumption of chocolate.[17]

Despite this, I caution against allowing a medical review worthy of inclusion in an evening news report tempt you to dash down to the candy store! For now, we know that cocoa is fine, but the saturated fat, sugar, and calories found in milk chocolate may offset any benefits it contains. Like any sugary food, you should only eat milk chocolate in moderation.

Heart Procedures

> For the life of the flesh is in the blood.
>
> —LEVITICUS 17:11

Leviticus contains Old Testament ceremonial laws. In chapter 17 God emphasizes the importance of blood. This chapter makes it clear that He required the Israelites to use great deference in handling blood, particularly the blood of a sacrificial animal. Why? The blood of the sacrifice had a grave and solemn purpose: atoning for sin, paying its penalty (death), and reestablishing fellowship with God. Because of this monumental purpose, God gave lengthy instructions on the process for the sacrifice—including who should perform it, where, how to select the animal, and what to do with the blood. The remainder of verse 11 quoted above reads, "And I have given it [blood] to you upon the altar to make atonement for your souls; for it is the blood that makes atonement for the soul."

This verse shows how blood represents life, physically and spiritually. All the organs and systems within our body are necessary for our existence; thus far we have only duplicated the kidneys' functions mechanically, through dialysis. Blood is the most symbolic substance when we consider life and death. Maybe this is because, unlike the other organs, blood moves, flows, and changes. This is much like humankind—during our lifetimes we move, flow, and change. Throughout our lives, blood transports needed components to every body part. Whether a platelet to curtail bleeding, a hormone to regulate metabolism, a white blood cell to fight infection, or oxygen to drive the whole operation—whatever is needed, blood delivers.

When circulation is blocked or compromised in any body part, the vulnerable tissue experiences *ischemia*, which means it is getting insufficient blood (and oxygen). Depending on the duration of the ischemia, either death or injury may ensue to the vulnerable tissue or the entire body. When atherosclerosis occludes coronary arteries, one of several possibilities can take place. If the blockage is chronic, mild ischemia stimulates the growth of new blood vessels (or enlargement of existing ones) to supply blood to the heart from an alternate route. This process is called "collateral circulation." Chronic stable angina may result when demand for blood temporarily exceeds the supply, such as if a person experiences a higher-than-normal amount of physical or emotional stress that overburdens the heart. In this instance, symptoms like pain or shortness of breath develop, prompting the person to relax (reducing demand), which restores the supply-and-demand curve back to its baseline.

However, if high demand persists, collateral circulation is not sufficient, or if a plaque ruptures and an occlusion quickly develops, an acute coronary syndrome (ACS)—either unstable angina or a myocardial infarction—may occur. With an ACS the main objective is restoring blood flow (the sooner, the better). A physician establishes a diagnosis by taking the patient's history to determine things such as the nature of the pain, its onset, associated symptoms, and the presence or absence of risk factors for cardiovascular disease. He also finds out whether the patient has suffered a previous heart attack or stroke. An electrocardiogram and blood tests help to confirm the diagnosis.

The physician may also administer oxygen and such medications as aspirin, nitroglycerin, morphine, beta-blockers, or statins and then decide how to best restore blood circulation. Depending on the circumstances, this can be done chemically through medications that will "dissolve" the occlusion (fibrinolysis) or a procedure. The two procedures I will review are:

♥ Coronary artery bypass graft surgery (or CABG, pronounced "cabbage"), where the surgeon uses veins or arteries from another part of the body to bypass the blockage

♥ A less complicated percutaneous coronary intervention (PCI), where an instrument is introduced into
the artery through the skin ("per" = through; "cuta-
neous" = skin) to open the blocked vessel and maintain its patency through a stent

Coronary artery bypass graft surgery

In addition to aggressive lifestyle modifications, coronary artery
disease can be managed conservatively with medications or, for
lack of a better term, invasively through procedures like CABG and
PCI, with CABG being the more invasive of the two. Conventional
CAGB surgery requires that the surgeon split open the sternum
(breastbone) to gain access to the heart. Since the late 1990s spe-
cialists have developed somewhat less dramatic techniques, which
continue to advance and evolve.

In patients with stable angina, the goals of therapy are to alle-
viate pain, slow the progression of atherosclerosis, and prevent the
development of a myocardial infarction or sudden cardiac death.
While this can be achieved conservatively in some, for others the
symptoms of angina are not adequately alleviated by this approach.
Or there may be limitations to using medications because of such
issues as side effects or allergies. Such situations may require a
more invasive approach (CABG or PCI) to control the symptoms
of angina and improve the quality of life. However, for a majority
of patients, the rate of mortality remains the same with an invasive
approach as with more conservative medical therapy.

Still, a select group with stable angina experiences survival benefits with revascularization, whether through CABG or PCI. This
includes people with blockage in the left main coronary artery,
those with a significantly positive stress test, or when the function
of the heart's left ventricle is severely compromised. While under
many circumstances PCI has replaced CABG as the procedure of
choice, CABG is still preferred when there is diffuse atherosclerosis

involving three or more vessels (especially in diabetics) or if a large portion of the heart muscle is at risk.

In the case of unstable angina, immediate intervention with angiography and revascularization is best for patients who have such complications as shock, heart failure, persistent pain while resting, valve dysfunction, or an irregular heart rhythm. For others who don't have these complications, angiography and revascularization (if necessary) is usually performed within twenty-four hours. In select circumstances—when patients are clinically stable and deemed at low or intermediate risk for complications—it may be safe to delay an intervention and manage them (at least initially) with conservative care.

CABG is rarely the procedure of choice in the case of an acute myocardial infarction, where time is of the essence and restoration of blood flow crucial. Under a limited set of circumstances, a person may require an operation in the setting of an acute heart attack; however, fibrinolysis and PCI can be accomplished in a fraction of the time needed to perform a CABG. The latter requires mobilization of an operating room and a team of surgeons, anesthesiologists, nurses, and technicians.

Percutaneous coronary intervention

First used in the 1970s, percutaneous coronary artery procedures restore blood flow to the heart in less invasive manner than a CABG operation. In PCI a cardiologist inserts a catheter into the body, usually through the femoral artery located at the top of the thigh. The catheter extends all the way to the heart, where the specialist uses it to correct the blockage. The first procedure developed was the percutaneous transluminal balloon angioplasty (PTCA). This utilizes a balloon tip catheter, inflated at the site of the blockage and helping blood flow freely again. The major complication with PTCA is re-blockage, either soon after the procedure or as long as eight months later.

Over time doctors developed heart stents as a means of curtailing this problem. While still inflating the balloon, a stent is inserted into the vessel after the dilation to maintain patency. With stents came a significant reduction in complications. Acute closure dropped from 2–10 percent to less than 1 percent, and sub-acute closure (within a month of the procedure) dropped from 5 percent to 0.5 percent. In addition, after the introduction of stents fewer people experienced heart attacks as a direct consequence of the procedure.

All stents contain a metal base. However, the prototype consisted solely of metal and was quite appropriately called a "bare metal stent" (BMS—notice that nearly everything has an acronym). However, as with CABG surgery, technology evolved and advanced so that drug-eluting stents have essentially replaced bare metal ones. Although these newer stents contain metal, they are coated with a polymer that is mixed with a drug, which is released over time. The drug helps prevent reclosure of the blood vessel. During the procedure, medications like heparin are used to stop blood clots from forming. Afterward doctors prescribe anti-platelet medications (e.g., aspirin and clopidogrel), along with statins, since they improve long-term outcomes and reduce the rate of occlusion.

With an acute myocardial infarction, patients whose blood flow is reestablished through PCI or fibrinolysis have a significantly better outcome than those who are not re-perfused. Of these two choices, PCI leads to lower rates of recurrent heart attack and lower death rates, compared to fibrinolysis. However, this advantage hinges on several variables, including the availability of PCI, how much time has elapsed between the heart attack and intervention, and the risks compared to the benefits of undergoing the procedure in any given patient.

Invasive procedures have greatly improved survival among people with heart attacks and greatly improved quality of life of those with angina. Yet they do not replace the need for aggressive lifestyle modification, including a heart-healthy diet, regular exercise, weight loss, and smoking cessation. Neither do they replace the need to optimally control such risk factors as diabetes, hypertension, and dyslipidemia, which require long-term medication use. Many people get discouraged at the prospect of having to take medications and regularly visit a health care provider, often for an indefinite period of time. If that describes you, let me remind you about the difference attitude makes and the blessings that come from choosing an optimistic outlook. Instead of feeling discouraged about pills and office visits, be grateful such options exist. Even though heart disease remains the leading cause of death in the United States, it is certainly not the ominous challenge it was just a few generations ago. And for that, we should all be thankful.

CONCLUSION

W ITH BOOK PROPOSALS, PUBLISHERS REQUIRE AUTHORS to identify a "target population"—the specific type of individual or group they hope to reach. Their aim is not to exclude or discourage anyone from reading the book, but to ensure the text creates maximum impact on those who need it the most. Choosing a target population also helps the marketing and advertising teams direct their efforts to the appropriate group. Of course, I was no exception to this rule. So I designated adult Christian men and women with cardiovascular disease (or at risk for it) as my primary target. With the high prevalence of heart disease in adults, regardless of religion, this represented a broad objective. Still, a subset within this large group captured my heart and served as my greatest motivation. As you may have guessed, that subset is pastors.

Being married to one, I admire and profoundly respect pastors. I appreciate the work they do and their faithfulness. As I mentioned earlier, as a pastor's wife I have firsthand exposure to what is required and the sacrifices pastors make to serve the Lord. Besides my husband's messages, over the years I have been blessed to hear perhaps hundreds of other pastors deliver sermons. While their texts vary and each one has a unique style, their ultimate goal remains to present the gospel message of salvation through faith in Jesus. When they approach their conclusion, it is common to hear (especially among "old school" preachers) the words, "I would be remiss…" followed by an invitation to accept Christ's atoning sacrifice.

It is no accident that I concluded this book with a discussion of the significance of blood—and its importance in *supplying* our entire body with a sufficient amount, all delivered by a healthy heart. Without blood we would not survive. However, like a good preacher, I would be remiss if I did not leave non-pastoral readers with the reminder that blood can *save*, eternally as well as physically. Our physical life is temporary and depends on the blood pumped by our hearts. Where we spend eternity, however, depends on whether we have faith in the blood Jesus shed at Calvary. My greatest objective has been compelling all readers to look beyond the physical and consider the spiritual. In addition, I prayed that anyone who started reading this book without knowing the One who saves would arrive at the end having decided to place their faith in Him. If that describes you, God has answered my prayer and allowed me to accomplish my purpose. I would encourage you to seek out a member of my "target population." Find a pastor who loves, edifies, and teaches his congregation, a pastor who even now may be waiting to meet you.

I hope that *Spiritual Secrets to a Healthy Heart* has been a source of encouragement and motivation. I hope you are inspired to make lifestyle changes that will lower your risk for cardiovascular disease in all its manifestations. And I hope and pray that God continues to prosper you and give you strength.

—KARA DAVIS, MD
CHICAGO, ILLINOIS

NOTES

Introduction

1. D. Lloyd-Jones, R. J. Adams, T. M. Brown, et al., "Executive Summary: Heart Disease and Stroke Statistics—2010 Update: A Report From the American Heart Association," *Circulation* 121, no. 7 (February 23, 2010): 948–954.

Chapter 1
Nutrition

1. W. C. Willett, F. Sacks, A. Trichopoulou, et al., "Mediterranean Diet Pyramid: A Cultural Mode for Healthy Eating," *American Journal of Clinical Nutrition* 61, no. 6 (June 1995): 1402S–1406S.

2. Merriam-Webster.com, s.v. "locavore," http://www.merriam -webster.com/dictionary/locavore (accessed October 11, 2012).

3. P. N. Mitrou, V. Kipnis, A. C. Thiébaut, et al., "Mediterranean Dietary Pattern and Predictin of All-Cause Mortality in a U.S. Population: Results From the NIH-AARP Diet and Health Study," *Archives of Internal Medicine* 167, no. 22 (December 10/24, 2007): 2461.

4. F. Sofi, F. Cesari, R. Abbate, G. F. Gensini, and A. Casini, "Adherence to Mediterranean Diet and Health Status: Meta-Analysis," *BMJ* 337, no. 7671 (September 20, 2008): 1344a.

5. Data obtained from the Centers for Disease Control and Prevention, Behavioral Risk Factor Surveillance System (BRFSS), http:// www.cdc.gov/brfss/ (accessed October 11, 2012).

6. Goodarz Danaei, Eric L. Ding, Dariush Mozaffarian, Ben Taylor, Jürgen Rehm, Christopher J. L. Murray, and Majid Ezzati, "The Preventable Causes of Death in the United States: Comparative Risk Assessment of Dietary, Lifestyle, and Metabolic Risk Factors," *PLoS Medicine* 6, no. 4 (April 8, 2009): http://www.plosmedicine .org/article/info:doi/10.1371/journal.pmed.1000058?imageURI=info :doi/10.1371/journal.pmed.1000058.t008 (accessed October 11, 2012).

7. M. Ezzati, A. D. Lopez, A. Rodgers, S. Vander Hoorn, and C. J. Murray, "Selected Major Risk Factors and Global and Regional

Burden of Disease," *The Lancet* 360, no. 9343 (November 2, 2002): 1347–1360.

8. R. H. Ward, P. G. Chin, and I. A. M Prior, "Tokelau Island Migrant Study: Effect of Migration on the Familial Aggregation of Blood Pressure," *Hypertension* 2 (July/August 1980): I43–I54.

9. R. D. Mattes and D. J. Donnelly, "Relative Contributions of Dietary Sodium Sources," *Journal of the American College of Nutrition* 10, no. 4 (August 1991): 383–393.

10. Quanhe Yang, Tiebin Liu, Elena V. Kuklina, et al., "Sodium and Potassium Intake and Mortality Among US Adults: Prospective Data From the Third National Health and Nutrition Examination Study," *Archives of Internal Medicine* 171, no. 13 (July 11, 2011): 1183–1191.

11. "The Diet and All-Causes Death Rate in the Seven Countries Study," *The Lancet* 318, no. 8237 (July 11, 1981): 58–61.

12. R. Sinha, A. J. Cross, B. I. Graubard, M. f. Leitzmann, and A. Schatzkin, "Meat Intake and Mortality: A Prospective Study of Over Half a Million People," *Archives of Internal Medicine* 169, no. 6 (March 23, 2009): 562–571.

13. F. B. Hu, M. J. Stampfer, J. E. Manson, et al., "Dietary Fat Intake and the Risk of Coronary Heart Disease in Women," *New England Journal of Medicine* 337, no. 21 (November 20, 1997): 1491–1499.

14. P. R. Marantz, E. D. Bird, and M. H. Alderman, "A Call for Higher Standards of Evidence for Dietary Guidelines," *American Journal of Preventive Medicine* 34, no. 3 (March 2008): 234–240.

15. M. W. Gillman, L. A. Cupples, D. Gagnon, et al., "Protective Effect of Fruits and Vegetables on Development of Stroke in Men," *Journal of the American Medical Association* 273, no. 14 (April 12, 1995): 1113–1117; and E. B. Rimm, A. Ascherio, E. Giovannucci, D. Spiegelman, M. J. Stampfer, and W. C. Willett, "Vegetable, Fruit, and Cereal Fiber Intake and Risk of Coronary Heart Disease Among Men," *Journal of the American Medical Association* 275, no. 6 (February 14, 1996): 447–451.

16. M. A. Pereira, E. O'Reilly, K. Augustsson, et al., "Dietary Fiber and Risk of Coronary Heart Disease: A Pooled Analysis of Cohort Studies," *Archives of Internal Medicine* 164, no. 4 (February 23, 2004): 370–376.

17. Lisa Brown, Bernard Rosner, Walter W. Willett, and Frank M. Sacks, "Cholesterol-Lowering Effects of Dietary Fiber: A

Meta-Analysis," *American Journal of Clinical Nutrition* 69, no. 1 (January 1999): 30–42.

18. S. Krishnan, L. Rosenberg, M. Singer, et al., "Glycemic Index, Glycemic Load, and Cereal Fiber Intake and Risk of Type 2 Diabetes in U.S. Black Women," *Archives of Internal Medicine* 167, no. 21 (November 26, 2007): 2304–2309.

19. Q Sun, D. Spiegelman, R. M. van Dam, et al., "White Rice, Brown Rice, and Risk of Type 2 Diabetes in U.S. Men and Women," *Archives of Internal Medicine* 170, no. 11 (June 14, 2010): 961–969.

20. L. S. Gross, L. Li, E. S. Ford, and S. Liu, "Increased Consumption of Refined Carbohydrates and the Epidemic of Type 2 Diabetes in the United States; An Ecologic Assessment," *American Journal of Clinical Nutrition* 79, no. 5 (May 2004): 774–779.

21. Presented at the March 23, 2011, American Heart Association Nutrition, Physical Activity, and Metabolism Conference and 51st Cardiovascular Disease Epidemiology and Prevention Annual Conference in Atlanta, GA, by Matthew J. Feinstein, Donald Lloyd-Jones, Jeff Levin, and Daniel P. Sulmasy.

22. JoAnn E. Manson, Walter C. Willett, Meir J. Stampfer, et al., "Body Weight and Mortality Among Women," *New England Journal of Medicine* 333, no. 11 (September 14, 1995): 677–685.

Chapter 2
Physical Activity and Exercise

1. K. E. Powell and S. N. Blair, "The Public Health Burdens of Sedentary Living Habits: Theoretical but Realistic Estimates," *Medicine and Science in Sports and Exercise* 26, no. 7 (July 1994): 851–856.

2. P. D. Wood, W. Haskell, H. Klein, S. Lewis, M. P. Stern, and J. W. Farquhar, "The Distribution of Plasma Lipoproteins in Middle-Aged Male Runners," *Metabolism* 25, no. 11 (November 1976): 1249–1257.

3. R. S. Paffenbarger Jr., R. T. Hyde, A. L. Wing, and C. C. Hsieh, "Physical Activity, All-Cause Mortality, and Longevity of College Alumni," *New England Journal of Medicine* 314, no. 10: (March 6, 1986): 605–613; and S. N. Blair, H. W. Kohl III, C. E. Barlow, R. S. Paffenbarger Jr., L. W. Gibbons, and C. A. Macera, "Changes in Physical Fitness and All-Cause Mortality, a Prospective Study of Healthy and Unhealthy Men," *Journal of the American Medical Association* 273, no. 14 (April 12, 1995): 1093–1098.

4. US Department of Health and Human Services, *2008 Physical Activity Guidelines for Americans*, available at http://www.health .gov/PAGuidelines/pdf/paguide.pdf (accessed October 12, 2012). You can also view the *Healthy People 2020 Objectives* at http://www .healthypeople.gov/2020/topicsobjectives2020/default.aspx (accessed October 12, 2012).

5. C. P. Wen, J. P. Wai, M. K. Tsai, et al., "Minimum Amount of Physical Activity for Reduced Mortality and Extended Life Expectancy: A Prospective Cohort Study," *Lancet* 378, no. 9798 (October 1, 2011): 1244–1253.

6. I. M. Lee, C. C. Hsieh, and R. S. Paffenbarger Jr., "Exercise Intensity and Longevity in Men. The Harvare Alumni Health Study," *Journal of the American Medical Association* 273, no. 15 (April 19, 1995): 1179–1184.

7. C. E. Matthews, K. Y. Chen, P. S. Freedson, et al., "Amount of Time Spent in Sedentary Behaviors in the United States, 2003–2004," *American Journal of Epidemiology* 167, no. 7 (April 1, 2008): 875–881.

8. D. Umpierre, P. A. Ribeiro, C. K. Kramer, et al., "Physical Activity Advice Only or Structured Exercise Training and Association With HbA1c Levels in Type 2 Diabetes: A Systemic Review and Meta-Analysis," *Journal of the American Medical Association* 305, no. 17 (May 4, 2011): 1790–1799.

9. E. W. Gregg, R. B. Gerzoff, C. J. Caspersen, D. F. Williamson, and K. M. Narayan, "Relationship of Walking to Mortality Among U.S. Adults With Diabetes," *Archives of Internal Medicine* 163, no. 12 (June 23, 2003): 1440–1447.

10. J. A. Meyerhardt, E. L. Giovannucci, S. Ogino, et al., "Physical Activity and Male Colorectal Cancer Survival," *Archives of Internal Medicine* 169, no. 22 (December 14, 2009): 2102–2108.

11. E. B. Larson, L. Wang, J. D. Bowen, et al., "Exercise Is Associated With Reduced Risk for Incident Dementia Among Persons 65 Years of Age and Older," *Archives of Internal Medicine* 144, no. 2 (January 17, 2006): 73–81.

12. M. Teychenne, K. Ball, and J. Salmon, "Physical Activity and Likelihood of Depression in Adults: A Review," *Preventive Medicine* 46, no. 5 (May 2008): 397–411.

13. B. H. Marcus, A. E. Albrecht, T. K. King, et al., "The Efficacy of Exercise as an Aid for Smoking Cessation in Women: A

Randomized Controlled Trial," *Archives of Internal Medicine* 159, no. 11 (June 14, 1999): 1229–1234.

Chapter 3
Habits and Preferences

1. Federal Trade Commission, "Federal Trade Commission Cigarette Report for 2006," 2009, http://www.ftc.gov/os/2009/08/090812cigarettereport.pdf (accessed October 12, 2012).

2. R. Huxley and M. Woodward, "Cigarette Smoking as a Risk Factor for Coronary Heart Disease in Women Compared With Men: A Systemic Review and Meta-Analysis of Prospective Cohort Studies," *Lancet* 378, no. 9799 (October 8, 2011): 1297–1305.

3. E. H. Wagner and T. Groves, "Care for Chronic Diseases," *BMJ* 325, no. 7370 (October 26, 2002): 913–914.

4. National Center for Chronic Disease Prevention and Health Promotion, "Tobacco Use: Smoking and Secondhand Smoke," *CDC Vital Signs,* September 2010, http://www.cdc.gov/VitalSigns/pdf/2010-09-vitalsigns.pdf (accessed October 12, 2012).

5. US Department of Health and Human Services, *A Report of the Surgeon General: How Tobacco Smoke Causes Disease: The Biology and Behavioral Basis for Smoking-Attributable Disease, 2010: The Report,* http://www.surgeongeneral.gov/library/reports/tobaccosmoke/index.html (accessed October 12, 2012).

6. TobaccoFreeKids.org, "Toll of Tobacco in the United States of America," fact sheet, http://www.tobaccofreekids.org/research/factsheets/pdf/0072.pdf (accessed October 12, 2012).

7. C. Willi, P. Bodenmann, W. A. Ghali, P. D. Faris, and J. Cornuz, "Active Smoking and the Risk of Type 2 Diabetes: A Systemic Review and Meta-Analysis," *Journal of the American Medical Association* 298, no. 22 (December 12, 2007): 2654–2664.

8. F. M. Booyse and D. A. Parks, "Moderate Wine and Alcohol Consumption: Beneficial Effects on Cardiovascular Disease," *Journal of Thrombosis and Haemostasis* 86, no. 2 (August 2001); 517–528; and J. H. O'Keefe, K. A. Bybee, and C. J. Lavie, "Alcohol and Cardiovascular Health: The Razor-Sharp Double-Edged Sword," *Journal of the American College of Cardiology* 50, no. 11 (September 11, 2007): 1009–1014.

9. K. J. Mukamal, M. K. Jensen, M. Grønbaek, et al., "Drinking Frequency, Mediating Biomarkers, and Risk of Myocardial Infarction

in Women and Men," *Circulation* 112, no. 10 (September 6, 2005): 1406–1413.

10. M.Roerecke and J. Rehm, "Irregular Heavy Drinking Occasions and Risk of Ischemic Heart Disease: A Systematic Review and Meta-Analysis," *American Journal of Epidemiology* 171, no. 6 (March 15, 2010): 633–644.

11. Flávio Danni Fuchs, Lloyd E. Chambless, Paul Kieran Whelton, F. Javier Nieto, and Gerardo Heiss, "Alcohol Consumption and the Incidence of Hypertension: The Atherosclerosis Risk in Communities Study," *Hypertension* 37, no. 5 (May 2001): 1242–1250.

Chapter 4
Choose a "Happy" Heart

1. Institute of Medicine, "Health Literacy: A Prescription to End Confusion," Report Brief, April 2004, http://iom.edu/~/media/Files/Report%20Files/2004/Health-Literacy-A-Prescription-to-End-Confusion/healthliteracyfinal.pdf (accessed October 12, 2012).

2. ThinkExist.com, "Scott Hamilton Quotes," http://thinkexist.com/quotation/the_only_disability_in_life_is_a_bad_attitude/219108.html (accessed October 12, 2012).

3. The Quote Garden, "Quotations: Dare to Be Great!", http://www.quotegarden.com/be-great.html (accessed October 12, 2012).

4. The Happy Manager, "Happy Quotes: Because You Might as Well Be Happy!", http://www.the-happy-manager.com/tips/happy-quotes/ (accessed October 12, 2012).

5. BrainyQuote.com, "Samuel Johnson Quotes," http://www.brainyquote.com/quotes/authors/s/samuel_johnson_2.html (accessed October 12, 2012).

6. Great-Quotes.com, "Italian Proverb Quote," http://www.great-quotes.com/quote/394 (accessed October 12, 2012).

7. J. A. Singh, M. M. O'Byrne, R. C. Colligan, and D. G. Lewallen, "Pessimistic Explanatory Style: A Psychological Risk Factor for Poor Pain and Functional Outcomes Two Years After Knee Replacement," *Journal of Bone and Joint Surgery* (Britain) 92, no. 6 (June 2010): 799–806.

8. Robert R. Edwards, Tarek Kronfli, Jennifer A. Haythornthwaite, Michael T. Smith, Lynanne McGuire, and Gayle G. Page, "Association of Catastrophizing With Interleukin-6 Responses to Acute Pain," *Pain* 140, no. 1 (November 15, 2008): 135–144.

9. B. R. Grossardt, J. J. Bower, Y. E. Geda, R. C. Colligan, and W. A. Rocca, "Pessimistic, Anxious, and Depressive Personality Traits Predict All-Cause Mortality: The Mayo Clinic Cohort Study of Personality and Aging," *Psychosomatic Medicine* 71, no. 5 (June 2009): 491–500.

10. T. Maruta, R. C. Colligan, M. Malinchoc, and K. P. Offord, "Optimists vs. Pessimists: Survival Rate Among Medical Patients Over a 30-Year Period," *Mayo Clinic Proceedings* 75, no. 2 (February 2000): 140–143.

11. K. H. Pitkala, M. L. Laakkonen, T. E. Strandberg, and R. S. Tilvis, "Positive Life Orientation as a Predictor of 10-Year Outcome in an Aged Population," *Journal of Clinical Epidemiology* 57, no. 4 (April 2004): 409–414.

12. H. A. Tindle, Y. F. Chang, L. H. Kuller, et al., "Optimism, Cynical Hostility, and Incident Coronary Heart Disease and Mortality in the Women's Health Initiative," *Circulation* 120, no. 8 (August 25, 2009): 656–662.

13. J. D. Hansen, D. Shimbo, J. A. Shaffer, et al., "Finding the Glass Half Full? Optimism Is Protective of 10-Year Incident CHD in a Population-Based Study: The Canadian Nova Scotia Health Survey," *International Journal of Cardiology* 145, no. 3 (December 3, 2010): 603–604.

14. M. F. Scheier, K. A. Matthews, J. F. Owens, et al., "Dispositional Optimism and Recovery From Coronary Artery Bypass Surgery: The Beneficial Effects on Physical and Psychological Well-Being," *Journal of Personality and Social Psychology* 57, no. 6 (December 1989): 1024–1040.

15. M. F. Scheier, K. A. Matthews, J. F. Owens, et al., "Optimism and Rehospitalization After Coronary Artery Bypass Graft Surgery," *Archives of Internal Medicine* 159, no. 8 (April 26, 1999): 829–835.

16. Hermann Nabi, Markku Koskenvuo, Archana Singh-Manoux, et al., "Low Pessimism Protects Against Stroke: The Health and Social Support (HeSSup) Prospective Cohort Study," *Stroke* 41, no. 1 (January 2010): 187–190.

17. Susan A. Everson, George A. Kaplan, Debbie E. Goldberg, Riitta Salonen, and Jukka T. Salonen, "Hopelessness and 4-Year Progression of Carotid Atherosclerosis: The Kuopio Ischemic Heart Disease Rick Factor Study," *Arteriosclerosis, Thrombosis and Vascular Biology* 17, no. 8 (August 1997): 1490–1495.

Chapter 5
Stress and Anxiety

1. National Institute of Mental Health, "The Numbers Count: Mental Disorders in America," October 12, 2012, http://www.nimh.nih.gov/health/publications/the-numbers-count-mental-disorders-in-america/index.shtml#KesslerPrevalence (accessed October 15, 2012).

2. E. J. Martens, P. de Jonge, B. Na, B. E. Cohen, H. Lett, and M. A. Whooley, "Scared to Death? Generalized Anxiety Disorder and Cardiovascular Events in Patients With Stable Coronary Heart Disease: The Heart and Soul Study," *Archives of General Psychiatry* 67, no. 7 (July 2010): 750–758.

3. S. Yusuf, S. Hawken, S. Ounpuu, et al., "Effect of Potentially Modifiable Risk Factors Associated With Myocardial Infarction in 52 Countries (the INTERHEART Study): Case-Control Study," *Lancet* 364, no. 9468 (September 11–17, 2004): 937–952.

4. Lorenzo Ghiadoni, Ann E. Donald, Mark Cropley, et al., "Mental Stress Induces Transient Endothelial Dysfunction in Humans," *Circulation* 102, no. 20 (November 14, 2000): 2473–2478.

5. E. Falk, "Why Do Plaques Rupture?", *Circulation* 86, Supplement III (1992): 30–42.

6. D. H. Solomon, E. W. Karlson, E. B. Rimm, et al., "Cardiovascular Morbidity and Mortality in Women Diagnosed With Rheumatoid Arthritis," *Circulation* 107, no. 9 (March 11, 2003): 1303–1307; and S. Manzi, E. N. Meilahn, J. E. Rairie, et al., "Age-Specific Incidence Rates of Myocardial Infarction and Angina in Women With Systemic Lupus Erythematosus: Comparison With the Framingham Study," *American Journal of Epidemiology* 145, no. 5 (March 1, 1997) 408–415.

7. T. Dietrick, M. Jimenez, E. A. Krall Kaye, P. S. Vokonas, and R. I. Garcia, "Age-Dependent Associations Between Chronic Periodontitis/Edentulism and Risk of Coronary Heart Disease," *Circulation* 117, no. 13 (April 1, 2008): 1668–1674.

8. D. O. Adams, "Molecular Biology of Macrophage Activation: A Pathway Whereby Psychosocial Factors Can Potentially Affect Health," *Psychosomatic Medicine* 56, no. 4 (July–August 1994): 316–327.

9. Mary F. Dallman, Susanne E. laFleur, Norman C. Pecoraro, Francisca Gomez, Hani Houshyar, and Susan F. Akana, "Minireview: Glucocorticoids—Food Intake, Abdominal Obesity, and Wealthy Nations in 2004," *Endocrinology* 145, no. 6 (June 2004): 2633–2638.

10. I. Kawachi, G. A. Colditz, A. Ascherio, et al., "Prospective Study of Phobic Anxiety and Risk of Coronary Heart Disease in Men," *Circulation* 89, no. 5 (May 1994): 1992–1997.

11. R. A. Kloner, J. Leor, W. K. Poole, and R. Perritt, "Population-Based Analysis of the Effect of the Northridge Earthquake on Cardiac Death in Los Angeles County, California," *Journal of the American College of Cardiology* 30, no. 5 (November 1, 1997): 1174–1180.

12. J. S. Steinberg, A. Arshad, M. Kowalski, et al., "Increased Incidence of Life-Threatening Ventricular Arrhythmias in Implantable DeFibrillator Patients After World Trade Center Attack," *Journal of the American College of Cardiology* 44, no. 6 (September 15, 2004): 1261–1264.

13. O. L. Shedd, S. F. Sears Jr., J. L. Harvill, et al., "The World Trade Center Attack: Increased Frequency of Defibrillator Shocks for Ventricular Arrhythmias in Patients Living Remotely From New York City," *Journal of the American College of Cardiology* 44, no. 6 (September 15, 2004): 1265–1267.

14. Y. J. Akashi, D. S. Goldstein, G. Barbaro, and T. Ueyama, "Takotsubo Cardiomyopathy: A New Form of Acute, Reversible Heart Failure," *Circulation* 118, no. 25 (December 16, 2008): 2754–2762.

15. Roland Rosmond and Per Björntorp, "Occupational Status, Cortisol Secretory Pattern, and Visceral Obesity in Middle-Aged Men," *Obesity Research* (now known as Obesity) 8, no. 6 (September 2000): 445–450.

16. R. Karasek, D. Baker, F. Marxer, A. Ahlbom, and T. Theorell, "Job Decision Latitude, Job Demands, and Cardiovascular Disease: A Prospective Study of Swedish Men," *American Journal of Public Health* 71, no. 7 (July 1981): 694–705.

17. R. Peter, J. Siegrist, J. Hallqvist, C. Reuterwall, T. Theorell, and the SHEEP Study Group, "Psychosocial Work Environment and Myocardial Infarction: Improving Risk Estimation by Combining Two Complementary Job Stress Models in the SHEEP Study," *Journal of Epidemiology and Community Health* 56, no. 4 (April 2002): 294–300.

18. Kristina Orth-Gomér, Sarah P. Wamala, Myriam Horsten, Karin Schenck-Gustafsson, Neil Schneiderman, and Murray A. Mittleman, "Marital Stress Worsens Prognosis in Women Woth Coronary Heart Disease: The Stockholm Female Coronary Risk Study,"

Journal of the American Medical Association 284, no. 23 (December 20, 2000): 3008–3014.

19. Linda C. Gallo, Wendy M. Troxel, Lewis H. Kuller, Kim Sutton-Tyrrell, Daniel Edmundowicz, and Karen A. Matthews, "Marital Status, Marital Quality, and Atherosclerotic Burden in Postmenopausal Women," *Psychosomatic Medicine* 65, no. 6 (November 1, 2003): 952–962.

20. James A. Blumenthal, Andrew Sherwood, Michael A. Babyak, et al., "Effects of Exercise and Stress Management Training on Markers of Cardiovascular Risk in Patients With Ischemic Heart Disease: A Randomized Controlled Trial," *Journal of the American Medical Association* 293, no. 13 (April 6, 2005): 1626–1634.

21. Mats Gulliksson, Gunilla Burell, Bengt Vessby, Lennart Lundin, Henrik Toss, and Kurt Svärdsudd, "Randomized Controlled Trial of Cognitive Behavioral Therapy vs. Standard Treatment to Prevent Recurrent Cardiovascular Events in Patients With Coronary Heart Disease, Secondary Prevention in Uppsala Primary Health Care Project (SUPRIM)," Figure 2, *Archives of Internal Medicine* 171, no. 2 (January 2011): 134–140. Used by permission.

22. Gulliksson, Burell, Vessby, Lundin, Toss, and Kurt Svärdsudd, "Randomized Controlled Trial of Cognitive Behavioral Therapy vs. Standard Treatment to Prevent Recurrent Cardiovascular Events in Patients With Coronary Heart Disease, Secondary Prevention in Uppsala Primary Health Care Project (SUPRIM)."

Chapter 6
Depression

1. World Health Organization, *World Health Statistics 2007*, Global Health Observatory, http://www.who.int/gho/publications/world_health_statistics/2007/en/ (accessed October 15, 2012). For the latest update, see http://www.who.int/gho/publications/world_health_statistics/en/index.html (accessed October 15, 2012).

2. M. Cepoiu, J. McCusker, M. G. Cole, M. Sewitch, E. Belzile, and A. Ciampi, "Recognition of Depression by Non-Psychiatric Physicians—a Systematic Literature Review and Meta-Analysis," *Journal of General Internal Medicine* 23, no. 1 (January 2008): 25–36.

3. W. J. Katon, "Clinical and Health Services Relationships Between Major Depression, Depressive Symptoms, and General Medical Illness," *Biological Psychiatry* 54, no. 3 (August 1, 2003): 216–226.

4. J. M. Donohue and H. A. Pincus, "Reducing the Societal Burden of Depression: A Review of Economic Costs, Quality of Care and Effects of Treatment," *Pharmacoeconomics* 25, no. 1 (2007): 7–24.

5. S. Moussavi, S. Chatterji, E. Verdes, A. Tandon, V. Patel, and B. Ustun, "Depression, Chronic Diseases, and Decrements in Health: Results From the World Health Surveys," *Lancet* 370, no. 9590 (September 8, 2007): 851–858.

6. Brett D. Thombs, Eric B. Bass, Daniel E. Ford, et al., "Prevalence of Depression in Survivors of Acute Myocardial Infarction," *Journal of General Internal Medicine* 21, no. 1 (January 2006): 30–38.

7. R. M. Carney and K. E. Freedland, "Depression, Moratality and Medical Morbidity in Patients With Coronary Heart Disease," *Biological Psychiatry* 54, no. 3 (August 1, 2003): 241–247.

8. M. A. Whooley, P. de Jonge, E. Vittinghoff, et al., "Depressive Symptoms, Health Behaviors, and Risk of Cardiovascular Events in Patients With Coronary Heart Disease," *Journal of the American Medical Association* 300, no. 20 (November 26, 2008): 2379–2388.

9. S. Win, K. Parakh, C. M. Eze-Nliam, J. S. Gottdiener, W. J. Kop, and R. C. Ziegelstein, "Depressive Symptoms, Physical Inactivity and Risk of Cardiovascular Mortality in Older Adults: The Cardiovascular Health Study," *Heart* 97, no. 6 (March 2011): 500–505.

10. S. J. Motivala, "Sleep and Inflammation: Psychoneuroimmunology in the Context of Cardiovascular Disease," *Annals of Behavioral Medicine* 42, no. 2 (October 2011): 141–152.

11. S. Wassertheil-Smoller, S. Shumaker, J. Ockene, et al., "Depression and Cardiovascular Sequelae in Postmenopausal Women. The Women's Health Initiative (WHI)," *Archives of Internal Medicine* 164, no. 3 (February 9, 2004): 289–298.

12. I. Connerney, R. P. Sloan, P. A. Shapiro, E. Bagiella, and C. Seckman, "Depression Is Associated With Increased Mortality 10 Years After Coronary Artery Bypass Surgery," *Psychosomatic Medicine* 72, no. 9 (November 2010): 874–881.

13. R. Churchill, M. Khaira, V. Gretton, et al., "Treating Depression in General Practice: Factors Affecting Patients' Treatment Preferences," *British Journal of General Practice* 50, no. 460 (November 2000): 905–906.

14. A. M. White, G. S. Philogene, L. Fine, and S. Sinha, "Social Support and Self-Reported Health Status of Older Adults in the

United States," *American Journal of Public Health* 99, no. 10 (October 2009): 1872–1878.

15. N. A. Christakis and J. H. Fowler, "The Spread of Obesity in a Large Social Network Over 32 Years," *New England Journal of Medicine* 357, no. 4 (July 26, 2007): 370–379.

16. I. Kawachi, G. A. Colditz, A. Ascherio, et al., "A Prospective Study of Social Networks in Relation to Total Mortality and Cardiovascular Disease in Men in the USA," *Journal of Epidemiology and Community Health* 50, no. 3 (June 1996): 245–251.

17. J. M. Cyranowski, T. L. Hofkens, H. A. Swartz, and P. J. Gianaros, "Thinking About a Close Relationship Differentially Impacts Cardiovascular Stress Responses Among Depressed and Nondepressed Women," *Health Psychology* 30, no. 3 (May 2011): 276–284.

18. J. H. Fowler and N. A. Christakis, "Dynamic Spread of Happiness in a Large Social Network: Longitudinal Analysis Over 20 Years in the Framingham Heart Study," *British Medical Journal* 337 (December 4, 2008).

Chapter 7
Curbing Anger

1. J. E. Williams, C. C. Patton, I. C. Siegler, M. L. Eigenbrodt, F. J. Nieto, and H. A. Tyroler, "Anger Proneness Predicts Coronary Heart Disease Risk: Prospective Analysis From the Atherosclerosis Risk in Communities (ARIC) Study," *Circulation* 101, no. 17 (May 2, 2000): 2034–2039.

2. I. Kawachi, D. Sparrow, A. Spiro III, P. Vokonas, and S. T. Weiss, "A Prospective Study of Anger and Coronary Heart Disease. The Normative Aging Study," *Circulation* 94, no. 9 (November 1, 1996): 2090–2095.

3. R. B. Shekelle, M. Gale, A. M. Ostfeld, and O. Paul, "Hostility, Risk of Coronary Heart Disease, and Mortality," *Psychosomatic Medicine* 45, no. 2 (May 1983): 109–114.

4. P. P. Chang, D. E. Ford, L. A. Meoni, N. Y. Wang, and M. J. Klag, "Anger in Young Men and Subsequent Premature Cardiovascular Disease: The Precursors Study," *Archives of Internal Medicine* 162, no. 8 (April 22, 2002): 901–906.

5. M. C. Cohen, K. M. Rohtla, C. E. Lavery, J. E. Muller, and M. A. Mittleman, "Meta-Analysis of the Morning Excess of Acute

Myocardial Infarction and Sudden Cardiac Death," *American Journal of Cardiology* 79, no. 11 (June 1, 1997): 1512–1516.

6. M. A. Mittleman, M. Maclure, J. B. Sherwood, et al., "Triggering of Acute Myocardial Infarction Onset by Episodes of Anger. Determinants of Myocardial Infarction Onset Study Investigators," *Circulation* 92, no. 7 (October 1, 1995): 1720–1725.

7. J. Moller, J. Hallqvist, F. Diderichsen, T. Theorell, C. Reuterwall, and A. Ahlbom, "Do Episodes of Anger Trigger Myocardial Infarction? A Case-Crossover Analysis in the Stockholm Heart Epidemiology Program (SHEEP)," *Psychomatic Medicine* 61, no. 6 (November–December 1999):842–849.

Chapter 8
Eden Is Over

1. V. L. Roger, A. S. Go, D. M. Lloyd-Jones, et al., "Heart Disease and Stroke Statistics—2011 Update: A Report From the American Heart Association," *Circulation* 123, no. 4 (February 1, 2011): e18–e209. Available online at http://circ.ahajournals.org/content/123/4/e18.full.pdf (accessed October 18, 2012).

2. Amy L. Arnold, Kerry A. Milner, and Viola Vaccarino, "Sex and Race Differences in Electrocardiogram Use (the National Hospital Ambulatory Medical Care Survey)," *American Journal of Cardiology* 88, no. 9 (November 1, 2001); 1037–1040; and Joan B. Lehmann, Paulette S. Wehner, Christoph U. Lehmann, and Linda M. Savory, "Gender Bias in the Evaluation of Chest Pain in the Emergency Department," *American Journal of Cardiology* 77, no. 8 (March 15, 1996): 641–644.

3. "Multiple Risk Factor Intervention Trial: Risk Factor Changes and Mortality Results," *Journal of the American Medical Association* 248, no. 12 (September 24, 1982): 1465–1477.

4. Jeremiah Stamler, Deborah Wentworth, and James D. Neaton, "Is Relationship Between Serum Cholesterol and Risk of Premature Death From Coronary Heart Disease Continuous and Graded?: Findings in 356,222 Primary Screenees of the Multiple Risk Factor Intervention Trial (MRFIT)," *Journal of the American Medical Association* 256, no. 20 (November 28, 1986): 2823–2828.

5. J. W. Rich-Edwards, J. E. Manson, C. H. Hennekens, and J. E. Buring, "The Primary Prevention of Coronary Heart Disease in

Women," *New England Journal of Medicine* 332, no. 26 (June 29, 1995): 1758–1766.

6. J. A. Cutler, P. D. Sorlie, M. Wolz, T. Thom, L. E. Fields, and E. J. Roccella, "Trends in Hypertension Prevalence, Awareness, Treatment, and Control Rates in United States Adults Between 1988–1994 and 1999–2004," *Hypertension* 52, no. 5 (November 2008): 818–827.

7. Administration of Aging, "Aging Statistics," US Department of Health and Human Services, http://www.aoa.gov/aoaroot/aging_statistics/index.aspx (accessed October 18, 2012).

8. N. M. Kaplan, "Primary Hypertension: Pathogenesis," in *Kaplan's Clinical Hypertension,* 9th ed., K. M. Kaplan, editor (Philadelphia: Lippincott, Williams and Wilkins, 2006), 50–121.

9. R. O. Halperin, H. D. Sesso, J. Ma, J. E. Buring, M. J. Stampfer, and J. M. Gaziano, "Dyslipidemia and the Risk of Incident Hypertension in Men," *Hypertension* 47, no. 1 (January 2006): 45–50.

10. D. I. Jalal, G. Smits, R. J. Johnson, and M. Chonchol, "Increased Fructose Associates With Elevated Blood Pressure," *Journal of the American Society of Nephrology* 21, no. 9 (September 2010): 1543–1549.

11. Aram V. Chobanian, George L. Bakris, Henry R. Black, et al., "The Seventh Report of the Joint National Committee on Prevention, Detection, Evaluation, and Treatment of High Blood Pressure: The JNC 7 Report," *Journal of the American Medical Association* 289, no. 19 (May 21, 2003): 2560–2571.

12. Centers for Disease Control and Prevention, "Number of Americans With Diabetes Rises to Nearly 26 Million," press release, January 26, 2011, http://www.cdc.gov/media/releases/2011/p0126_diabetes.html (accessed October 19, 2012).

13. Rochester General Health System, "Type 1 Diabetes," http://www.rochestergeneral.org/centers-and-services/rochester-general-medical-group/services/diabetes/about-diabetes/types-of-diabetes/type-1-diabetes/ (accessed October 19, 2012).

14. Centers for Disease Control and Prevention, "Number of Americans With Diabetes Rises to Nearly 26 Million."

15. Ibid.

16. Ibid.

17. R. D. Brook, B. Franklin, W. Cascio, et al., "Air Pollution and Cardiovascular Disease: A Statement for Healthcare Professionals From the Expert Panel on Population and Prevention Science of the

American Heart Association," *Circulation* 109, no. 21 (June 1, 2004): 2655–2671.

18. R. D. Brook, S. Rajagopalan, C. A. Pope III, et al., "Particulate Matter Air Pollution and Cardiovascular Disease: An Update to the Scientific Statement From the American Heart Association," *Circulation* 121, no. 21 (June 1, 2010): 2331–2378.

Chapter 9
Medications and Procedures

1. Centers for Disease Control and Prevention, "High Blood Pressure: High Blood Pressure Facts," October 17, 2012, http://www.cdc.gov/bloodpressure/facts.htm (accessed October 19, 2012).

2. C. Baigent, A. Keech, P. M. Kearney, et al., "Efficacy and Safety of Cholesterol-Lowering Treatment: Prospective Meta-Analysis of Data From 90,056 Participants in 14 Randomised Trials of Statins," *Lancet* 366, no. 9493 (October 8, 2005): 1267–1278.

3. S. Singh, Y. K. Lioke, and C. D. Furberg, "Thiazolidinediones and Heart Failure: A Teleo-Analysis," *Diabetes Care* 30, no. 8 (August 2007): 2148–2153.

4. C. L. Roumie, A. M. Hung, R. A. Greevy, et al., "Comparative Effectiveness of Sulfonylurea and Metformin Monotherapy on Cardiovascular Events in Type 2 Diabetes Mellitus: A Cohort Study," *Annals of Internal Medicine* 157, no. 9 (November 6, 2012): 601–610. The reason for the increased risk was not entirely clear, but these medications will certainly be the focus for future research to shed light on these findings.

5. J. M. Rapola, J. Virtamo, S. Ripatti, et al., "Randomised Trial of Alpha-Tocopherol and Beta-Carotene Supplements on Incidence of Major Coronary Events in Men With Previous Myocardial Infarction," *Lancet* 349, no. 9067 (June 14, 1997): 1715–1720; and J. M. Gaziano, J. E. Manson, and P. M. Ridker, et al., "Beta-Carotene Therapy for Chronic Stable Angina," *Circulation* 94, suppl I (1996): 508.

6. E. R. Miller III, R. Pastor-Barriuso, D. Dalal, R. A. Riemersma, L. J. Appel, and E. Guallar, "Meta-Analysis: High-Dosage Vitamin E Supplementation May Increase All-Cause Mortality," *Annals of Internal Medicine* 142, no. 1 (January 4, 2005): 37–46.

7. E. Lonn, S. Yusuf, M. J. Arnold, et al., "Homocysteine Lowering With Folic Acid and B Vitamins in Vascular Disease," *New England Journal of Medicine* 354, no. 15 (April 13, 2006): 1567–1577.

8. R. D. Jackson, A. Z. LaCroix, M. Gass, et al., "Calcium Plus Vitamin D Supplementation and the Risk of Fractures," *New England Journal of Medicine* 354, no. 7 (February 16, 2006): 669–683.

9. M. J. Boland, A. Grey, A. Avenell, G. D. Gamble, and I. R. Reid, "Calcium Supplements With or Without Vitamin D and Risk of Cardiovascular Events: Reanalysis of the Women's Health Initiative Limited Access Dataset and Meta-Analysis," *British Medical Journal* 342 (April 19, 2011).

10. Evangelos C. Rizos, Evangelia E. Ntzani, Eftychia Bika, Michael S. Kostapanos, and Moses S. Elisaf, "Association Between Omega-3 Fatty Acid Supplementation and Risk of Major Cardiovascular Disease Events: A Systematic Review and Meta-Analysis," *Journal of the American Medical Association* 308, no. 10 (September 12, 2012): 1024–1033.

11. F. M. Sacks, A. Lichtenstein, L. Van Horn, et al., "Soy Protein, Isoflavones, and Cardiovascular Health: An American Heart Association Science Advisory for Professionals From the Nutrition Committee," *Circulation* 113, no. 7 (February 21, 2006): 1034–1044.

12. D. J. Becker, R. Y. Gordon, S. C. Halbert, B. French, P. B. Morris, and D. J. Radar, "Red Yeast Rice for Dyslipidemia in Statin-Intolerant Patients: A Randomized Trial," *Annals of Internal Medicine* 150, no. 12 (June 16, 2009): 830–839.

13. O. Weingärtner, M. Böhm, and U. Laufs, "Controversial Role of Plant Sterol Esters in the Management of Hypercholesterolaemia," *European Heart Journal* 30, no. 4 (February 2009): 404–409.

14. P. J. Mink, C. G. Scrafford, L. M. Barraj, et al., "Flavonoid Intake and Cardiovascular Disease Mortality: A Prospective Study in Postmenopausal Women," *American Journal of Clinical Nutrition* 85, no. 3 (March 2007): 895–909.

15. S. Kuriyama, T. Shimazu, K. Ohmori, et al., "Green Tea Consumption and Mortality Due to Cardiovascular Disease, Cancer, and All Causes in Japan: The Ohsaki Study," *Journal of the American Medical Association* 296, no. 10 (September 13, 2006): 1255–1265.

16. D. J. Maron, G. P. Lu, N. S. Cai, et al., "Cholesterol-Lowering Effect of Theaflavin-Enriched Green Tea Extract: A Randomized Controlled Trial," *Archives of Internal Medicine* 163, no. 12 (June 23, 2003): 1448–1453.

17. A. Buitrago-Lopez, J. Sanderson, and L. Johnson, et al., "Chocolate Consumption and Cardiometabolic Disorders: Systematic Review and Meta-Analysis," *British Medical Journal* 343 (August 26, 2011).

INDEX

FINALLY...
a Permanent Weight-Loss Solution

This easy-to-follow 50-day plan emphasizes both the physical and spiritual aspects of healthy living, inspiring positive habits that help you lose weight and keep it off for good. It's time to let God work a miracle in you!

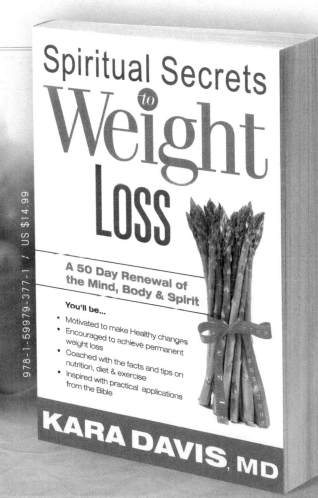

AVAILABLE AT BOOKSTORES,
online, and in e-book

SILOAM

11377

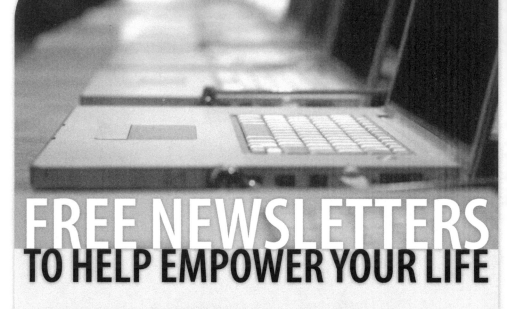

FREE NEWSLETTERS
TO HELP EMPOWER YOUR LIFE

Why subscribe today?

- ❏ **DELIVERED DIRECTLY TO YOU.** All you have to do is open your inbox and read.

- ❏ **EXCLUSIVE CONTENT.** We cover the news overlooked by the mainstream press.

- ❏ **STAY CURRENT.** Find the latest court rulings, revivals, and cultural trends.

- ❏ **UPDATE OTHERS.** Easy to forward to friends and family with the click of your mouse.

CHOOSE THE E-NEWSLETTER THAT INTERESTS YOU MOST:

- Christian news
- Daily devotionals
- Spiritual empowerment
- And much, much more

SIGN UP AT: **http://freenewsletters.charismamag.com**

8178